THE BODY IMAGE BLUEPRINT

Your Go-To Guide for
Radical Self-Reverence

JENNY EDEN BERK, MSEd

THE BODY IMAGE
BLUEPRINT

Your Go-To Guide for
Radical Self-Reverence

JENNY
EDEN BERK, MSEd

CONTENTS

I am deeply grateful for my mom and dad for supporting me in everything I do and inspiring me to pursue my passions. To my amazing husband and three children, for tolerating long days of me obsessively typing away at my computer, sometimes at the expense of a decent dinner. To Abby, for shepherding me to continue my body-positive path when I desperately wanted to give up, and for giving me the courage to do our photoshoot. To Everett and everyone at Gymnasia, for showing me how much joy I could get from moving my body. Special thank you to Kathy Wheeler, whose beta course, The 90 Day Book, pushed me to finally write the book of my dreams. All of your support has been immeasurable.

"To be beautiful means to be yourself. You don't need to be accepted by others. You need to accept yourself."

—THICH NHAT HANH

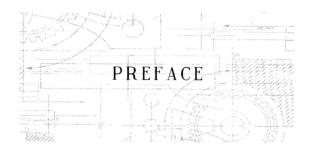

PREFACE

I have always been fascinated with accounts of near-death experiences. So many of these stories are the same: A highlight reel of their life, a deep sense of love and oneness, the ability to hover over their body, and a great pulling sensation toward a beautifully alluring light. Whether or not you choose to believe these accounts as a sign of a spiritual higher power or simply a hallucination in a dying person's mind to help cope with death, it is striking to hear how there are central themes of love, comfort, acceptance, and a separation of soul and body. In one woman's story that I recently read, she talked about how she had always felt so confined to her body and that it didn't feel like it even belonged to her. When she had her near-death experience, she felt that her soul was the only thing that had mattered, not the "space suit" she embodied on Earth. When she was revived, she devoted the rest of her life to tapping into that soul to allow its light to affect others. I was struck by that notion. I wondered what it would be like if we could all feel our identity more within our souls rather than the exterior shell that encapsulates us on Earth. Would we feel free? Would we feel happier?

I think about women who have battled breast cancer and lost a part of their identity with the loss of their breasts. I've thought about men and women who feel they were born into the wrong body. I've even thought about those who lose or gain a large amount of weight and can no longer identify with what is now presented to them in the mirror. Are all of these people, in a sense, having a near-death experience? Are they "reborn" into an exterior they can accept and appreciate by recognizing that it merely houses the beautiful soul inside?

This is deep stuff, but I think about all the suffering that human beings endure when thinking about their bodies. I wonder how we can connect more with our inner selves so we are able to express on the outside the love and light that is inherently inside. Can we nurture our souls by feeding our bodies nourishing and comforting foods? Can we move our bodies in ways that make us feel strong and happy so that we can manifest our gifts to the world in the deepest ways possible? Can we connect souls to other souls the same way we connect physical bodies to other bodies? It seems daunting amid all the external noise, media, and magazines that promulgate the idea that our exterior package matters more.

I am able to separate mind and body when I'm meditating or when I'm in any body of water. I enjoy the glorious, weightless feeling that lifts me to the surface no matter what I weighed that morning on the scale. This is unmatched by any other experience I have had. I wonder if this kind of sensory separation is partly what inspires astronauts to launch into space. Beyond the obvious science and extraterrestrial curiosity, are they also longing to reach that higher plane, that sense of weightlessness, or a near-death experience?

We may never have answers to all of these complex questions, but what I do know is that rather than aggressively trying to change our exteriors in order to be loved and accepted, we must begin consciously tuning into our interiors. We need to tap into that light to be able to give more on Earth in the short time we have here. Only when we connect with our souls, with our true essence and with the essence of others, will we be able to experience Heaven on Earth.

IN DIETS WE TRUST

We live in a diet-centric world. Girls are indoctrinated at a young age by family, peers, and society to dutifully subscribe to the false notion that beauty resides in some subjective prescribed size. The many that comply often find themselves in a messy web of chronic dieting, over-exercising, and body-loathing. They bully their bodies relentlessly until they reach this perceived "Shangri-La" weight, and then are faced with the notion that either they are still not happy or that they lack an exit plan and skills to help them keep this weight off in a healthy and sustainable way. This begins the dejá vu dieting cycle.

This book is about jettisoning the notion that we are not good enough as we are. It's about finding ways to systematically fight the patriarchal system—be it from media, peers, family, or even ourselves—that tells us we cannot ever be worthy of happiness unless we fit a predetermined mold. My personal blueprint begins by telling you my story as that is what informs everything else that follows. My story of indoctrination into, and ultimately separation from, the chronic dieting world underscores the pain that millions of other little girls and boys experience with their own identity every day. The ways I conformed to dieting culture at times, and girded against it at others, will hopefully be accessible and valuable to you. The stories I will share in Part 2 of this book will be relatable yet heartbreaking at times. We will all find pieces of ourselves in these stories. They come from many women and men who I have interviewed over the past six months. The patterns of pain, shame, and insecurities about our bodies that emerge are at once remarkable in their rawness and unremarkable because of the commonality between them.

A blueprint is a detailed plan, a course of action, and I seek to provide that for you. Part 3 of this book is your personal blueprint for going from a body-basher to basking in body-reverence. It is devoted to the very techniques, tools, and strategies I employed to heal my own body image and the ones that I use with my clients every day to help them find a healthy, balanced, and joyful approach to eating, exercising, and appreciating their bodies. This is not a quick fix self-help book, but rather it is the beginning of a path; a path I want to explore with you. At times, it will be circuitous, bumpy and difficult, but ultimately, this path can lead you to a place of peace and happiness you never thought was possible with respect to your body image. I urge you to take this journey with me.

PART I
MY BLUEPRINT

"What lies behind us and what lies before us are tiny matters compared to what lies within us."

—RALPH WALDO EMERSON

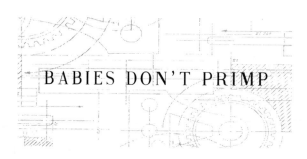

BABIES DON'T PRIMP

Humans are born with an innate sense of embodiment. Babies move around, marveling at their kinesthetic abilities, large and small, and practice these new accomplishments as often as possible. My own babies would relinquish sleep in lieu of standing up and sitting back down in their cribs over and over again, much to my chagrin. Babies begin to earnestly strive for movement and new physical abilities with each passing day. I would watch for hours as my children attempted and finally accomplished lifting their heads, rolling over, getting up on all fours, crawling, standing up, walking, and eventually running! It's all such a beautiful, miraculous process.

Toddlers are unabashed in their nakedness and they absolutely delight in their various body parts, learning what feats they can accomplish with those parts. They also love to show off their new skills like squatting, bending down to touch their toes, somersaulting, and jumping into puddles. They know how amazing the human body is without having to intellectually process it. They just want to use it and they feel so much innate pride in doing so.

Sadly, somewhere along the way to adulthood, this sense of wonder and appreciation comes to an abrupt halt. For many, it is replaced with shame and loathing and a desperation to change what is on the outside in order to satisfy the false notion that only by fitting into a predetermined mold on the outside will a person know love, worthiness, and acceptance.

Like many girls and boys, this was my sad trajectory as well.

I can't say that I remember the "golden" years of running around naked and feeling free and unabashed in my skin, but if you ask my parents, that was my truth and it was abundant. There is, in fact, an impressive bounty of photographic evidence showcasing this joyful nudity. I seemed to be naked all the time!

As a child, I was very open and expressive. I would happily greet everyone with a smile and I talked to strangers without hesitation. I didn't have an unusual childhood, except perhaps that it was unusually ordinary. No major drama, life event, illness, or trauma happened along the way that could be easily pinpointed as the thing that broke my spirit and nudged me in the direction of body loathing and excessive dieting. My parents were consistent pillars of love and acceptance in my life, always present and dynamic sources of life's greatest energies. My mom, a wonderful, smart and caring woman, bent over backwards to help me become a resilient, kind, and confident person. My dad, with whom I share a very close relationship, was also instrumental in helping me know that I am deserving of unconditional love. I was and am very lucky to have had them build the foundation in my life that has ultimately brought me so many blessings and success.

My mom's career as a gourmet chef meant our after-school snacks were no joke—this was not some apples and peanut butter situation. I am talking full-blown, mouthwatering hors d'oeuvres on the daily. I can recall coming home from school to find my mother experimenting with making pastries in the shape of a swan with a glorious pool of ganache to swim upon—the kind of stuff snack-happy kids' dreams are made of. The downside of this was that I was the only one in my family who struggled with their weight, so while other people in my family could take or leave these delicacies, I often felt compelled to chow down on them fast and furiously.

My mom is a petite woman, yet always talked about her own struggles with weight and body image. It was hard for me to summon sympathy about that given her small frame, and I often felt she couldn't possibly know what it was like to truly struggle. However, like many of us, our perceptions of ourselves are vastly different than those around us and I cannot, in good conscience, deny her experience of herself despite the fact that I felt there was no way she could possibly understand my plight.

She also worked hard to help me develop a healthy relation-ship with food, from teaching me to slow down and to sit down when I ate to helping me tune into when I was hungry. I give her full credit for my absolute love of vegetables because she lovingly and expertly cooked them every day for us.

Apparently, I have always been loud and proud regarding my love for food. My dad remembers me at a mere eighteen months old, sticking my hand out of the crib, which was my locally famous sign for, "More chocolate milk in my baba (bottle) please!" Yep, even as a baby, I made it known that chocolate and sweets were right up my alley. There was even that time when upon watch-ing my mom throw out an entire roll of cookie dough in horror,

I furtively and gingerly fished it out of the trash when she wasn't looking and kept it in my closet for a week, eating it at my leisure. It's an actual miracle that I didn't get salmonella!

The truth is that girls don't fish cookie dough out of a trash can "George Costanza style" unless there are some serious food issues going on. One of the phases of dieting indoctrination is this idea that some foods are good and others are bad. And yes, if you eat the broccoli then you are good, but if you dare eat the Twinkie, well, you might as well have punched a nun. What I know now and impart to others is that food is not moral. Food is merely energy that makes our bodies feel and function differently depending on the type of food. Yes, I fell prey to this "good food/ bad food" phenomena that is often a precursor to years of binging and restricting and yo-yo dieting.

Let me make this clear. I don't blame my parents. They simply wanted my brother and me to be nourished and healthy. But, inadvertently, there was a dynamic trajectory set up in my home that allowed me to see food in moral terms and thus ascribe that morality to myself. This can be extremely damaging to one's body image and the trajectory of their relationship to food. I spend months in my practice helping people to recover from this sad cycle.

Trying to figure out the "why" as it pertains to the downward spiral of my own body image is a difficult task, but one worth attempting. There probably isn't one thing or one person or one incident to blame, and as I dig back through my childhood, there were definite signs that I was falling into a dark rabbit hole of negative body image.

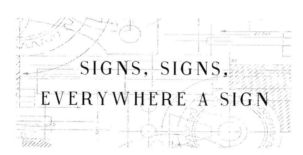

SIGNS, SIGNS, EVERYWHERE A SIGN

I remember feeling pretty good about myself for a little while. However, there were signs that told me I should believe otherwise. The comments made to us as young children can have devastating, lasting effects, even in what seem to be the most benign situations.

For instance, I remember having dinner with a friend and her family when I was nine years old. There were no restrictions, no diets, no embarrassment about my appetite back then. When I stopped eating the delicious meal her family had made for us, there was some food left on my plate, and I'll never forget what my friend's mom had to say about that.

"Jenny, you're not done eating, are you? You look like you must usually eat much more than this at home, right?"

Even as I recall this memory years later, I am flooded with the same humiliation. No, I did not normally eat much more than that. I ate when I was hungry and stopped when I was full the same way many human beings do, but in that split second, I was introduced to the concept that other people possibly perceived me as heavy, even though I didn't perceive myself that way, and that was devastating. Even at a young age, I felt stripped of my power and I began to question my reality. I favored the external perceptions and opinions of other people about my body more than my own, and it would only get worse with time.

DR. STRANGETUSH: HOW I LEARNED TO STOP WORRYING AND LOVE THE BUM

For as far back as I can remember, I've known that I am equipped with a distinctive backside. See this picture?

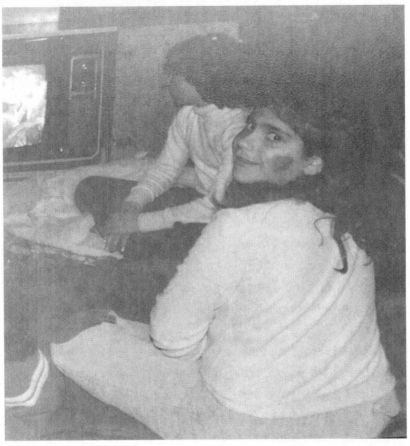

I think I am eight years old here and I clearly remember being self-conscious when the woman taking the photo told me to turn around. I thought, foolish as it may seem, that she was staring at my big butt.

This self-consciousness continued and grew for years. In junior high school, friends remember me never wanting to take off my bulky coat in the winter. I knew why, but didn't admit it at the time. I was ashamed of my body and ashamed of how big my bottom was and I wanted it covered at all times.

As I got older, this fear mitigated a bit as I slowly learned to hate other parts of my body as well. "Look at my huge thighs," or, "Wow, my arms are so fat!" were common mantras in my head, and I eventually shared them with friends. It almost didn't matter that my butt was big because everything else seemed to match it! Even though the booty positive anthem "Baby Got Back" was very popular at that time, I was intentionally oblivious to the benefits of a big booty.

It wasn't until Jennifer Lopez came onto the scene in the late nineties that I realized a distinctive booty was actually something that was considered sexy and beautiful; something that some men loved and women coveted!

You can imagine how floored I was when the butt lifter product came out into the market—an article of clothing that was made specifically to give women a bigger booty; something I had naturally yet spent most of my time loathing!

Nowadays, it's commonplace to see celebrities galore flaunting their "assets!" From Jennifer Lopez to Kim Kardashian, it's everywhere you look. We even have the fabulous Meghan Trainor singing that it's "ALL about that bass."

I am not going to say that I don't still have days where I feel self-conscious about my tush and the way it seems to have an identity all its own, but I can say that I have grown comfortable in my skin and have learned to love my hourglass shape. Just as importantly, I also love the power and strength that I have built in my rear from doing squats, single leg deadlifts, and kettlebell swings! It may be large, but it is also noticeably in charge.

I even recently overcame my self-doubt and modeled in the nude for a photographer friend who specializes in artistic nudes. This was extremely hard for me to do but very healing and freeing at the same time. My friend, who shot a bunch of my backside, certainly showcased a part of me that I had never seen or considered in a positive light before. So now, instead of the constant negative self-talk and self-consciousness, I focus on the wise words of Sir Mix-a-Lot: "So Cosmo says you're fat? Well, I ain't down with that. You can do side bends or sit-ups, but please don't lose that butt!"

Okay, Sir Mix-a-Lot. If you say so.

Now, when I see this picture of me, I want to crawl back in time and hug that little girl and tell her that her tush is beautiful and that this woman just wants to take a nice, completely harmless picture of her. I want to tell her that her beauty is inherent and to please never doubt herself.

THE GREAT TABLE EXPERIMENT

I recall going to a lot of themed activity parties when I was in elementary school—video game parties, makeup parties, even a specific baton twirling party. Who knew that was a thing? Anyway, it was at a roller-skating party in fourth grade where I came to realize that my weight was indeed different than other girls my age and not just some hypersensitivity in my mind.

I was finishing up roller-skating and decided to sit on one of the tables nearby to take my skates off. I hopped up on the table and, much to my chagrin, the table actually bent and came off its hinges! Thankfully, no one noticed, but I was mortified and ashamed that my pre-adolescent body weight was able to do that.

Quickly, I fixed the table, putting it back on its hinges. I scanned the room, looking for someone else that this might happen to if they sat on the table. I found a girl at the party who I thought was around the same size as me and asked her to sit on the same exact table too. She stared back at me, obviously bewildered as to why the heck I would ask her to do this. I couldn't tell her why. It was my own little super sleuth body image experiment that I had to get to the bottom of. For whatever reason, she obliged and jumped up onto the table backwards. Nothing happened. No movement, no hinges breaking, not even a little weight-induced creak. Nothing!

I was crushed. This was the first time I realized that my perception of myself compared to what other people saw were two very different things. I imagined that my size was the same as this girl's when, clearly, I was larger and heavier. I was only ten at the time, but this experience shaped me for years to come and added to my own confusion about how I looked, making me question my ability to trust in my reality.

HELLO MUDDAH, HELLO FADDAH

We often adopt our perceptions of body image directly from our parents, mostly without even knowing it. As little girls, we look to our mothers to see how they treat themselves, how they view their own bodies. We start to build ideas about what it means to value ourselves as well as what it means to not value ourselves. We look to our fathers for affirmation, whether we mean to or not, and we subconsciously know whether they value our mother's worth or not.

Problems in this familial system arise when we function within a patriarchal system that sets up expectations for what makes women valuable. When our mothers begin to question their worth because the media says they're not skinny enough, the insecurities this creates in our mothers are transposed onto us. When our mothers diet and worry about portion control, we subconsciously adopt that same complicated relationship with food.

My mother knew nothing of dieting when she was growing up. My grandmother hadn't lived in a time when women's bodies were subject to such deep scrutiny as they are now. But when weight-loss programs and dieting fads began to pop up in the early eighties, my mom was subconsciously swept up in the trends of her time. All of a sudden, everyone's moms were dieting, all of her friends were worried about their waistlines, and dieting became part of the collective vernacular. There wasn't any reason to be wary of this shift in trend, and the women of my mother's generation had no warning about the psychological impact this cultural shift would have.

Like any tradition, dieting and body image are inadvertently passed down through the generations, and though my mom bent over backwards to try and not make food an emphasis, it was too late. Society had already made me feel that I wasn't ideal, and through no fault of her own, this perception was validated by my mom's own perception of body image. We were both victims of the patriarchy.

This is why I decided to stop dieting. I made a conscious decision to cut off the blood supply to body image insecurities built upon patriarchal fallacies so that future generations, my daughters, have a chance at a more positive sense of self. Because, for me, growing up with such embedded insecurities made things more painful than they should've been, and though she tried, my mother couldn't solve it for me.

In the summer before middle school, I had an amazing opportunity to go to "sleep away" camp. Like other girls afforded the same experience, I relished in the enjoyment of doing arts and crafts, swimming, horseback riding, skiing, and sharing a bunk with seven other exuberant girls from the tri-state area. I bonded particularly well with my counselors and looked up to them the way any young girl looks up to whomever she perceives to be cooler and older than she.

You might imagine how sad it made me that while other girls my age got piggy back rides to and from the mess hall, my options were limited to hand-holding or arm-hooking. The counselors tried to give me piggy back rides but their struggle was obvious and it was far too humiliating to let them keep trying. Yet again, I stood confronted with the heartbreaking fact that I was larger than my peers and that this kept me from the simple yet coveted joys of a young girl's life, like piggy back rides from her favorite camp counselor. I don't recall the moment exactly, but at some point during my time at sleep away camp, young as I was, I felt strongly for the first time that I needed to do something about my weight.

I recently re-read some of the letters I sent home to my parents that summer. Many are just normal, happy letters recalling the week's activities. I bragged of my skiing and swimming accomplishments, discussed my new friendships, and disclosed any juicy bunk drama. Other letters involved me begging and pleading to be picked up. (I think my exact words were, "Do you see that this letter is wet and smeared? That's because I'm crying and I need you to come get me RIGHT NOW!") That my parents refused to pick me up and left me to figure things out on my own is pretty remarkable to me, and I believe it is partially what built the resiliency I have in me today. And then, of course, there was the succession of letters listing exactly what I wanted them to bring for visiting day: Doritos, Reese's Peanut Butter Bars, Coke, gum, and new outfits for my Cabbage Patch Kid, Deidre, who, in case you were wondering, was, indeed, named after the *Days of Our Lives* character. There was one letter I came across, however, that absolutely crushed me. It's a ten-year-old me recalling the week's activities as usual, but I also describe some other things I was proud of.

"Mom! Dad! Guess what? The nurse weighed us in and I weighed ninety pounds! I lost a pound! Isn't that amazing? Also, I didn't eat the peanut butter at lunch. Are you proud of me?"

Typing these words now, as an adult, makes me emotional and teary. I want to jump back in time and hug that little girl and tell her to eat the damn peanut butter and to enjoy every bite. I want to tell her that she is loveable and worthy and beautiful just the way she is and that there is no need to try to lose weight at age ten. I want to hold her close and beg her to please not start down this dangerous, slippery path of dieting and restricting. But I can't. And maybe it's best that way.

Every experience I've had, every diet I've endured, every pound lost or gained brought me to the place I am now; to the place where I can proudly share my story, and more importantly, where I can hopefully help other girls to only stumble where I once fell. Without these experiences, I highly doubt I could be as effective as I am now at helping others heal from these deep wounds and develop a healthier, more sustainable relationship with food and their bodies. While incredibly painful to recall, I am grateful for these fundamental life events as they shaped me and gave me the depth and access to overcome challenges that now allow me to help other people with compassion and grit.

THE JUNIOR HIGH BLUES

I don't know of a single friend who remembers middle school as a happy time. I dare you to find one! No, in fact, most people I speak to recall middle school as a special kind of hell, highlighting that extremely awkward time in our lives where we were going through puberty and trying to navigate the murky social waters without a lifeboat. I got my period in sixth grade, developed breasts in seventh, and by eighth grade, I could be found lamenting that boys were not paying attention to me as much as

I had hoped they would. At only thirteen years old, I was already subscribing to the narrative that I would not be attractive to boys and no one would want to date me until I lost weight.

I wore an extremely garish and particularly bulky colorful winter coat in seventh grade, which would be fine except that I NEVER TOOK IT OFF. In fact, my best friends, many of whom I am still close with to this day, remember me sitting in class, awkwardly trying to push up the sleeves of this coat like one would do with a long-sleeved shirt if they were getting warm. The coat didn't even come off during lunch time. My mom would balk at the various food items smeared on my precious coat each day, unaware that these were actually painful vestiges of my once healthy body image. I thought I was being coy—*no one can see or notice my enormous booty if I wear this coat, right?* I'd be fashionably hidden under massive amounts of strange, puffy eighties material so as to bamboozle anyone who might consider me bigger than the other girls my age. What I didn't realize at the time was how sad, pathetic, and awkward I must have looked in that big ugly coat. Ahhh, middle school. It's fine. Just call me Puff Daddy.

During recess one day, two older girls, disguised as my friends, approached me on the field while I pretended to be doing something social (I was probably just twiddling my thumbs). They had a plan. The plan was to embarrass me under the guise that they were being helpful and supportive. Each shouting one word at a time, they spewed out, "We! Think! You! Should! Wear! A! Bra!"

There it was. Just like that, my boobs were on display, spotlighted by the crass environment that only exists on a middle school playground. I was wildly flustered, but also defiant and defensive, "I am wearing a bra, stupid!" Ironically, I had just started wearing one that week. You can imagine the shame and discomfort I felt the rest of the day knowing that my budding little micro boobs were the topic of conversation on the playground that day. I started to long for my winter coat after that little episode, even though it was full on spring at that point. The extra layer metaphorically protected me from both the vast changes that were going on externally while also cushioning my deeper feelings of insecurity and shame that were starting to bubble to the surface.

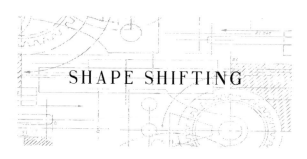

SHAPE SHIFTING

B y fifteen, I was full-on dieting. Weight Watchers was my first attempt. My family encouraged me but were also very careful to make it more about my health, not just my weight. I should mention at this juncture that I was only 140 pounds, but to me, this was wildly unacceptable. I also tried the Cabbage Soup Diet, The Scarsdale Diet (I was from Scarsdale after all), and my own low-fat, low-carb diet using a book to help me count my fat grams and carbs. Of course, the diets were always coupled with my consistent daily overdose of exercise in the form of intense ninety-minute step aerobics followed by a strength training class followed by a long walk home.

When I confronted my mom as an adult about why I had such poor body image and why I felt the need to diet at such a young age, she recalled that I was miserable and relentlessly begged her to take me to Weight Watchers. To a degree, I believe this to be true. I know I was greatly affected by my peers and by the reality that I was, indeed, heavier than most of my friends. My body image fiasco was also bolstered by the belief that I would never have a boyfriend or have anyone find me attractive unless I was very thin.

It is also true that my pediatrician had mentioned on more than one occasion that I ought to consider a diet to get me into a more acceptable BMI range. All of that said, I can't help but feel that my family, specifically my mom, played a big role in the development of my body image as well. It's not that she was at all blatant about this. My mom supported and loved me no matter my size and only wanted me to be happy. She felt great consternation that I was in emotional pain about my size and felt stymied about how to help me feel better. I think a big part of the problem was that my mom, albeit unintentional, affected me with her own insecurities about her own size and appearance.

It was my mom's own dieting indoctrination, her constant fascination with diets and actual dieting, along with the comments I'd overhear her say about other people's bodies that slowly infiltrated and crafted my delicate belief systems about appearance and self-worth. Even though I could not intellectually process it at the time, and even though this message was subtle and often deliberately concealed (the last thing my mom would have wanted was for me to be insecure about my body), I still received the message loud and clear. Thin was important. Appearance was everything. Dieting and restricting were the means to thinness and acceptable appearance. This is the setting in which many of us begin our journey toward obsessive dieting. I hear it all of the time from my clients.

Make no mistake. Our media's promulgation of an ideal beauty standard and the influence of our peers deeply affect us as well, but this internal struggle for external perfection often begins in the home with our families and, most often, our mothers, with whom we consciously and unconsciously try to emulate.

I was also first diagnosed with hypothyroidism at fifteen. This is a significant detail because while I cannot solely blame Hashimoto's thyroiditis for my inability to maintain a smaller body, it certainly didn't do me any favors, and I came to understand that it would always be a struggle to have the thinner body that I wanted. What I didn't know is that I would have to literally bully my body with extreme dieting and punishing exercise just to maintain a body weight I wasn't satisfied with in the first place. I didn't know that I'd be setting myself up for a lifetime of chronic dieting and the polarities of binging and restricting. To be clear, I had no idea of the detrimental effects of ongoing restrictive diets on my body, my metabolism, and my psyche. The hypothyroidism only made me more determined that I would stop at nothing to be the size I wanted. I just had to work harder.

The final provocation came in the car while I was complaining to a trusted friend about my weight and what seemed to be an inability to lose it fast enough in time for a rendition of the play *Little Shop of Horrors*. I'd been cast as one of the doo-wop girls and had to perform in an extremely tight dress. I was 135 pounds and absolutely hated my body. I refused to put on the skin-tight dress for the performance. My friend casually said to me while driving, "Jenny, I hate to see you so miserable, and if you are really unhappy, you can consider getting liposuction someday." I bristled and felt completely deflated and angry. I promised myself on that day that I would never, ever resort to getting fat sucked out of my body by some machine while I lay unconscious in a hospital bed.

I remember sorting all of this out in my mind—alternately plotting my next diet and how I could exercise enough to lose ten pounds in time for the show, and despite my previous revulsion, actually entertained the idea of what liposuction would look and feel like. The easy way out did seem appealing at times, but no, I would never do that. Even at eighteen, I was falling prey to competing voices in my head. One said, "No! You don't need to resort to liposuction! You are fine the way you are," and the other more domineering voice always said things like, "It's time to restrict. It's time to burn more calories. You won't be successful or have a boyfriend or be lovable or attractive until you do this." It was these two competing voices that would follow me well into adulthood and permeate every aspect of my life, even my career.

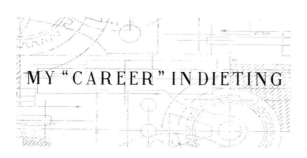

MY "CAREER" IN DIETING

My twenties were all about finding myself and my passions—who did I want to be when I grew up? I tried working at "cool" companies like New York Magazine, Universal Records, and New Line Cinema. I did, in fact, finally start dating and had several relationships throughout my twenties while living in NYC. Those were relatively good times. I felt carefree and happy with only intermittent bouts of dieting and self-loathing.

When I started dating one man, however, he happened to be friends with a previous boyfriend who I overheard warning him that my weight "fluctuated a lot." Can you imagine warning someone about this as if it was on par with cheating or being a compulsive liar? "You better be careful about dating that Jenny character. She's nice and loyal and funny and all, but man, her weight fluctuates a lot!" This is the body-conscious, beauty-obsessed, weight-focused culture we live in.

After some dalliances in the media and music world, I decided it was time to pursue a helping field, which I felt was much more suited to my natural skillset and inclinations. I have always been fascinated by psychology and by human behavior so I decided to get my master's degree at the University of Pennsylvania for Psychological Services in the School of Education. I found an internship working in the Health Education department at the university and ended up conducting intake sessions with students, running drinking prevention programs, and honing my communication and life coaching skills.

And then it happened...

I met my husband. Finally, after years of worrying whether I would ever have a boyfriend to then wondering if I would ever find "the one," he showed up in the most organic way. We met at a party while I was visiting Boston from Philly. We had both gone to the same college and graduated the same year and found out we have a tremendous amount in common. The only bad part? He lived in Boston and I was still finishing up my internship and research job in Philly. Six months later, I moved to Boston to be with him.

I started job searching the second I arrived and was so fortunate to find an amazing career very quickly at a national health and weight management company as a health educator. I facilitated classes and worked one-on-one with patients going through a very rigorous, medically supervised weight management program. The interview process was intense and long, spanning many weeks and many steps, but when I was finally hired, I truly felt I was on a path that was just right for me.

I ended up working at this company for thirteen years. I got engaged and married during my tenure there. I grew and birthed three children while working there. This company played a pivotal role in my life and in my career. There were patients I worked with for over ten years, developing meaningful and powerfully effective coaching techniques that would support their overall health and wellness, and for some, the strategies I helped implement actually gave them their lives back. Being able to play a role in that process gave me immeasurable joy and satisfaction. My passion for working intimately with people was finally coming to fruition. My co-workers were very special and caring human beings and I believed deeply in the company's values and tenets. I totally drank the proverbial Kool-Aid.

I was very happy there, learning the ropes and working with patients. One of the values of the company was to have staff act as role models of health for our clients by practicing the very health behaviors we would teach our patients to carry out. That included writing in a food log, eating lots of fruits and vegetables, and using the company's meal replacements. As a vegetarian of fifteen years, there were some limitations to the pre-packaged entrees they produced that I could eat, but to be honest, the ones I could eat sort of ignited my gag reflex. *How did I go from eating pastry swans in a pool of ganache to this crap?* But I wanted to be a dutiful employee and follow the rules. Therefore, I forced myself to eat these meals despite my strong aversion to them. I did enjoy the line of smoothie products they produced so I happily drank those with no problem.

I had been an employee for roughly three to six months when I walked in one morning and my manager asked to have a sit-down meeting with me. *Could I have done something wrong?* I had been getting fabulous feedback up until this point from both clients and staff, yet my hands were sweaty walking into her office. She looked a bit flustered but jumped right in. She went on to explain that being a good role model was one of the values of the company and asked if I would consider doing one of the company's signature weight loss programs, replete with at least two of those horrid pre-packaged meals. I was flabbergasted. *Was my boss seriously asking me to lose weight for my job? Is that even legal?*

I vacillated between feeling ashamed and recalcitrant, much like I had felt many other times in my life when faced with either conforming to dieting pressure or defying it. My manager had not asked me to do this in a bubble. This had apparently come from higher up in the company. She reminded me that I had assured them during my interview that I would work toward being a good role model, and that doing one of the diets to get to a "healthy" weight was a wonderful way to inspire our patients. To be honest, I was devastated. I didn't know whether to quit on the spot or show her what a good little dieter I could be. These thought processes all went on within the two seconds I had to spare before responding. Defiance won out initially, "...But, I am an excellent role model." I went on, "I eat healthy with lots of fruits and vegetables as my staples, I exercise regularly, and I practice yoga and meditation." My biometrics were also excellent with very low cholesterol, perfect blood pressure, and no underlying health issues aside from the hypothyroidism. If I wasn't the picture of good health, I didn't know what was. Apparently, my 150-pound frame was way too heavy to be considered a healthy weight and I was left reeling.

According to the antiquated and much maligned (from my perspective) BMI scale, at my height of 5'3", I needed to be 139 pounds or under in order to be considered in the healthy range. I was, in fact, "overweight." I knew very little, if anything, about the Health at Every Size movement at this point in my life and I trusted other people or experts more than I trusted myself. I ultimately decided to comply and got to work on my new diet right away.

DIETING 2.0

Along with my dignity, I lost fifteen pounds on my work-prescribed diet, and truth be told, as hard as it was, I was definitely enjoying my more svelte body and the way it fit into some clothes that I had tucked deep in the back of the closet, namely my *Little Shop of Horrors* doo-wop costume.

The problem, of course, was that I had no exit plan after this dieting experience. I was exerting about 800 calories of exercise daily and taking in about 1200 calories. I had starved myself down enough to fit into my wedding dress, which had been strategically altered in anticipation of me losing weight. This was my main motivation, of course, because a 150-pound bride was, for me, clearly unacceptable. After all that work, I still berated myself for not being able to get even skinnier.

Despite my disappointment with my body, our wedding day was the best day of my life. Our subsequent honeymoon to Australia was spectacular as well. With my newly minted weight loss, I had the stamina to walk all over the country, snorkel, and participate in a scary but fun bridge walk in Sydney. While we were in Cairns, near the Great Barrier Reef, my new husband and I decided to go parasailing together. I put the harness on and got all ready for the adventure when the outfitter for the parasailing company made an off-handed remark that I might be too big to get up in the air. All the wind got sucked out of me in that moment and, once again, I was filled with shame and embarrassment.

The fact that my husband was right there to witness this made it all the more humiliating. *Are you kidding me?* I was 135 pounds, and not only that, I had worked my mother-loving tush off just to get to this "too large" of a body to get up during parasailing. *Was this person completely out of touch? Was he mocking me? Was he truly concerned for me? Am I really being body shamed on my own damn honeymoon?* Luckily for all of us, I had no problem being hoisted in the air, and the hubby and I had a wonderful time together. As I had done so many times before, I sucked the comment deep inside of me and forgot about it, all the while knowing I'd plot my next restrictive diet as soon as I got home.

Losing all the weight was wonderful and I felt great, *but was it enough to make that lifestyle sustainable?* Of course it wasn't. As it had always done before, the weight crept back on slowly and insidiously. I gained six pounds on my honeymoon alone—a by-product of the extreme restriction I had endured just prior to my wedding. My body was dying to get some weight back on and was screaming for me to just eat! The honest truth is, when one pushes for quick weight loss, as I had always done before, it's a form of bullying your body and will almost always result in your body eventually rebelling—raising your metabolic set point and setting you back for the long haul.

THE BODY BULLY

Everyone hates a bully, right? A bully is someone who tries to exert control over one or more people by taunting, insulting, intimidating, or verbally abusing them. We talk about bullies in school, on the playground, and even in politics. The overarching idea is that bullies basically "suck" and we should not tolerate any bullying under any circumstances.

Yet, it's those same people who despise and reprimand bullies that often bully themselves! Imagine Biff Tannen from *Back to the Future* yelling at and berating you non-stop. You wouldn't tolerate that (hopefully) and you would take action! So, why don't we take action against our own negative attacks?

The problem is that when it's you attacking yourself, who can report it? What tactics can you possibly use?

A few years ago, I went to the gym seeking to simply notice the number of times I said something negative about myself when looking in the mirror. Things like, "You should be stronger by now," or, "Ugh, you look pregnant in that Lululemon top," or, "I can't compete with these women in this class!" are all examples of little thought bubbles that appeared without warning. After an hour of a down-and-dirty workout (which was supposed to make me feel strong and empowered), I had counted eighteen times in which I thought something negative about my body or my abilities! Eighteen times!! Can you imagine if you insulted someone else you love eighteen times in one hour? That person would probably never talk to you again, yet we do it to ourselves day-in and day-out, relentlessly.

We bully by denying or judging our appetite. We bully by going on restrictive and unsustainable diets. We bully by refusing to listen to our bodies, and we bully by using exercise as punishment for eating something fattening as opposed to moving for the joy of it. We bully by constantly berating our physical appearance, creating a chronic low level stress response in our bodies, which signals our bodies to create inflammation, decreases muscle mass, and increases fat storage. These are all things we do not want! In fact, I believe that much of the malaise, allergies, autoimmune disorders, and GI distress that Americans have today are partly attributable to the stress of bullying our bodies in this way.

Can we agree to finally start a truce and befriend our bodies? If you were to write a letter to your body, what would you say? Could you say, "I'm sorry," and raise the white flag? What would happen if when you caught yourself attacking you turned it around and said something kind instead? What if you even "fake it till you make it?"

I know this has worked for me. I "thought-stop" in the moment whenever I catch myself talking trash about myself. I thought-stop, turn it around, and even when it's the last thing I am feeling or wanting to say, I find something kind to say and find one thing to be grateful for.

Let's all agree to stop mean-girling and Biff-Tannening our bodies. Do it for your mental wellbeing as well as for your overall path to physical and emotional wellness.

I bullied my body relentlessly into a shape and size it didn't want to be naturally for the next thirteen years. Where dieting was once solely driven by my own insecurities and body-loathing, now there was a palpable external pressure coming in the form of my company as well. It was a double whammy of feeling the urgent need to be thin and all of the obsessive and heroic efforts put forth daily to be a good role model.

A LITTLE BIT PREGNANT

Only a mere six months after my husband and I got married, we were pregnant with our first daughter. We were so delighted, and I marveled at my ever-changing and growing baby bump. Morning sickness for the first twelve weeks precluded me from sticking with my high veggie and fruit diet in lieu of the more belly comforting options of toast, pizza, and crackers. So, I guess it won't be a shock to you when I tell you that I gained more than the suggested two to three pounds in my first trimester. It was actually more like eight to ten pounds and I knew I was in for a long nine months.

When a male OBGYN, subbing for my regular MD, saw me for one of my pregnancy visits, he said, "You know, you're gaining weight a bit fast for the first trimester." I think I actually whispered the words, "No shit, Sherlock," before nodding politely. I believed my body to be a weight gain machine and it did not disappoint! My pregnancy was like weight gain on steroids. It was like a train wreck I could see coming but was helpless to stop. Again, I was faced with the two polarities of myself. One side was busy relishing in the fact that I finally didn't have to diet. After all, I was growing a baby! On the other side, shame was my constant companion, especially as I got up in front of a room of people looking to me to help them lose weight, every day knowing I was doing the exact opposite. The pressure was intense, but I went about my life doing the best I could and kept working and teaching until the very day I went into labor.

Whereas my baby bump was cute, my post-baby bump was atrocious. Those stories you hear about women leaving the hospital in their pre-pregnancy jeans? Yeah, not so much for me. I think

I left in some stretchy puke green pajamas if I remember correctly. Ah, yes, the ones with the extra forgiving elastic waistband. The stories about how all my weight would just melt away because I was breastfeeding? That was a total myth for me as well. I was faced with the cold hard reality that the only way I could lose weight was to wait until I was finished breastfeeding (a year) and put in another full court press. And press I did.

For this post-partum dieting attempt, I used my company's program again, but this time, I had to do an 800 calorie per day diet for it to work at all. The weight came off but I was miserable, often light-headed, and always resentful. As luck would have it, the second I got to my goal weight of 139 pounds (the healthy weight as per BMI), I got pregnant and it all started again. Two more times in fact. I began to call the process "dejá vu dieting," because it had all started to feel so familiar, like I had been there before. I had.

DEJA VU DIETING

"I have been here before," you say. I remember eating this piece of celery with no dip and being starved in this very same spot before! I get this weird feeling that I've actually been on this treadmill before. Is there creepy cosmic stuff going on or is it just dejá vu dieting?

"What is dejá vu dieting?" you ask. It's the phenomenon of finding yourself in the same dieting situation year after year with no sustainable results. It's sometimes called the oh-crap-bathing-suit-season-is-coming-up-panic juice cleanse. It's the wow-$10-a-month-for-this-crappy-gym-is-a-steal-especially-since-I'll-only-go-once mentality.

The problem with dejá vu dieting is this: The definition of insanity is doing the same thing over and over and expecting a different result! Don't you want to get off that dieting roller coaster? There is a way. Let it all go. Seriously! Focus on quality nutritious food, eat for pleasure, savor your food, and be mindful of the process. Move your body in new and exciting ways. Embody your body. Appreciate the myriad of ways you can heal yourself through nourishing food. Take a scale hiatus and simply trust a little in your own body cues and wisdom.

Our default is to always go back to a black and white, extreme diet or binge mentality. We know that this doesn't work and often causes a higher set weight than before you dieted in the first place. This, in turn, makes the process an even higher uphill battle.

I always anticipated that I would gain weight during pregnancy and that it would be a challenge to lose it once I became a busy, tired mom. What I didn't anticipate, however, was that my baby bump would remain with me into eternity. I struggled at work. I was scared to wear empire waisted clothing for fear people would suspect I was pregnant. I dealt with questioning looks at my navel area and even the occasional, "When are you due?" Those comments were soul crushing. No one knew how hard I worked to be healthy and thin. The comments would at once motivate me to work harder and leave me depressed and resigned to utter failure.

When I finally was able to heal my relationship with my body for good, I came to accept this bump as beautiful evidence of growing my amazing babies, whom I now nurturing outside the womb to become caring, open, and non-judgmental people. This process took a long time. I think many of you, especially my mommy readers, are interested in a new, more novel approach to postpartum body image.

WHY I NOW LIKE IT WHEN SOMEONE ASKS ME WHEN I'M DUE

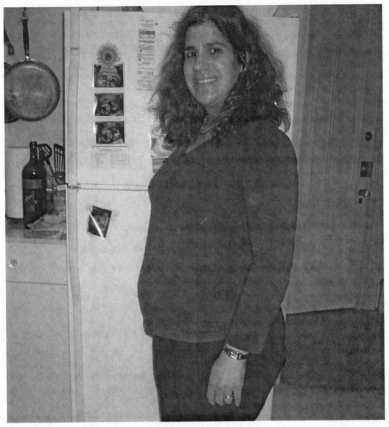

When I was a child, I remember sticking out my belly to see what I would look like if I were pregnant. Pretend-time with friends often included a ball under a shirt to play the part of the "pregnant mom." But when I actually became pregnant eleven years ago, I was self-conscious about the burgeoning "bump" and the possibility that people would notice it before I was ready to announce to friends and family that we were expecting a baby.

As the bump grew, I reveled in the attention I received, the knowing smiles from older women, and even the random strangers that wanted to touch my belly. I realized that, for many, pregnancy represents a joyous and exhilarating time of discovery, growth, and transition on many levels, even between strangers.

What I did not anticipate, however, was that six weeks AFTER my baby was born, people would still ask me, "When are you due?" Ouch! Give a girl a break! My uterus hadn't even had time to return to its original size yet. I had always known about the "post-bump" phenomenon, and even as a young adult, I could spot a woman who had given birth pretty easily. But after my daughter was born, I balked when my mom gave me the book *How to Lose Your Mummy Tummy*. As I had always had a rather flat belly, I didn't expect it to be an issue for me.

Not only was I dead wrong, but sadly, I discovered that despite heroic dieting efforts and diligent core strengthening exercises, the bump was apparently here to stay. This was only compounded when I got pregnant for the second and third time. In fact, I began showing with the third baby as soon as I saw the double line on the pee stick. Just joking! (Not really.)

At one point during what I'll call the "desperate years," I even consulted a plastic surgeon to see if I had a common condition called diastasis, where the muscles in the lower abdomen separate during pregnancy and fail to close back after the birth, causing a pouch effect in the tummy. "Nope," the MD said. "Your muscles are perfect and solid and in the right place, with just some extra skin and fat on top." Oh, okay, doc. Gotcha. Thanks...

The frequent comments of, "How far along are you?" and, "Wow! Are you going to have another baby?" caused me great consternation—to the point that I wanted to walk around with a sign saying, "No, I'm not pregnant, just bloated and a bit 'overweight,' but thanks!" Personally, I would never ask anyone that question unless I was 200% sure she was pregnant (e.g. seeing their water break in front of me or the baby crowning), but alas, many others do not seem to have the same level of sensitivity in this area. I've come to accept that and I don't begrudge their curiosity and attempts at friendliness.

Just recently, I've decided to take another approach. No, I didn't quadruple my efforts to undo the bump via diet and exercise, nor did I choose surgery. Instead, I decided to regard it as a COMPLIMENT when someone thinks that I look pregnant. Now, I think that it must be because I am glowing and that I must still look young enough for people to assume that I can get pregnant. Woohoo! Young, nubile, fertile, and glowing! Just what a 42-year-old woman wants to hear!

So, to all the pre-moms, pregnant ladies and post-moms, let's make peace with our bumps, shall we? Let's honor them, cherish them, and thank them for giving us the ability to create these incredible beings that we get to shape, mold, and turn into caring, sensitive human beings that hopefully won't ask random people on the street, "When are you due?" But next time someone asks you that question, be happy! Because it means you look like a badass, fertile, hot mama. Own it, girlfriend!

THE INTERNAL
METAMORPHOSIS

After twelve years of working with my company, I started to grow restless. I started to grapple with questions about whether I was truly helping people or merely putting a salve on their wounds without acknowledging or addressing the deeper issues that cause people to overeat in the first place. I started to feel guilty for prescribing restrictive diets and counseling people on how to stick to them when I knew deep down that, for most of them, it would only result in eventual weight regain, potentially leaving them sicker than when they first started, and without an exit plan. I started to wonder if there was more I could do in my career to help people get to the root cause of binge eating and emotional eating. By now, my children were getting older and more independent. Up until that point, I was fearful of pursuing a new direction with my career because of the flexibility my company offered me in terms of working part-time and having the ability to wear the mommy hat too—something that was very important to me when my children were small. I was also growing tired and frustrated by my own lack of ability to maintain weight once I had lost it. I was so incredibly tired of dejá vu dieting and desperately wanted to stop, but I was too afraid that if I let go of the reins, even a little bit, that the weight would pour on with no end in sight.

Simultaneously, I started to do extensive personal research on what might be wrong with my body given what a weight gain machine I perceived myself to be. I read books on autoimmune disease and Hashimoto's thyroiditis, I sampled bizarre supplements, tried cutting out artificial sweeteners, sugar, and processed foods. I went to a yoga retreat center to "detox" and learn mindful eating. I went to a variety of different doctors to see what my possible diagnosis could be. My research landed me in a functional medicine office where multiple hormonal, blood, urine, and saliva tests were conducted. The results? Leaky gut, multiple food sensitivities, and systemic inflammation from stress. I believed that my chronic dieting and body-bashing literally stressed me and my body so much that it caused my entire immune system to flare up, making it nearly impossible for me to lose weight. The worst part of this information was that it was recommended that I give up all gluten, dairy, tomatoes, and peanuts. Might I remind you that, at this point, I had already been a vegetarian for twenty-five years for ethical and environmental reasons. This additional restrictive protocol would prove to be just too much. I am a rule follower and I am deferential, possibly to a fault, especially toward medical experts, sometimes eschewing my own bodily wisdom in favor of what an outside "expert" had determined was best for me. Ten months and a gluten-free, vegan diet later, I was diagnosed with Orthorexia.

HOW GIVING UP GLUTEN MADE ME ORTHOREXIC

Orthorexia: An obsession with eating foods that one considers healthy to the point of extremes and to the detriment of one's psyche.

After a slew of tests revealed potential allergies to numerous foods, and as a vegetarian of twenty-six years, it seemed unfathomable that I would have to restrict my eating even more.

I'd already annoyed my friends and family enough by being the "picky" eater, but now, obsessed with the reasons why I couldn't lose weight despite my heroic efforts, sitting in a doctor's office, I was hearing that in order to reduce inflammation in my body and recover from leaky gut syndrome, I had to also give up gluten and dairy.

In my desperation to stay healthy and thin, I took on this great challenge and managed to persevere for ten months, but it came at a great cost to me physically, socially, and psychologically.

At first, I saw it as a challenge. I downloaded gluten-free restaurant-finder apps, created a Pinterest board devoted to gluten-free, vegan living and relentlessly researched all the foods I could eat and say "yes" to so that I wouldn't feel as deprived. It was hard, to be sure, but I was managing and also cooking a lot more at home to make the task a lot easier.

I had hoped for a dramatic change in the way I felt—more energy would've been nice, less brain fog sounded awesome, instant weight loss would have me elated, etc. The truth is, none of these things happened. In fact, the most important lesson was that I realized I did not have any symptoms to begin with! I felt exactly the same not eating gluten as I had eating it. Same for dairy, peanuts, tomatoes, and about fifteen other foods I had to omit to give this "allergy discovery" a fair shot.

I started to see certain foods, even healthy foods, as toxic to me. I became obsessed at restaurants that there be no cross-contamination. Friends and family started to worry about me and my commitment to this new protocol. It was one thing if I were seeing massive positive changes in how I felt, but yet another to actually feel more preoccupied and more anxious about food than ever before with no change whatsoever in my digestion and overall wellbeing.

It wasn't until some further testing showed I had an overgrowth of bacteria and needed to go on a strong dose of antibiotics that everything changed. The antibiotics made me so ill and nauseous that one day, at our neighborhood block party, I wolfed down almost half a pizza—all the gluten and dairy I could handle that day. After a few hours, I felt no change aside from being really full. Over the next few days, I tested the waters further by adding more and more gluten and dairy back into my diet. I felt so happy and so liberated. Best of all, I felt no change whatsoever in how my body felt on these foods. I realized that the food allergy/sensitivity diagnosis not only made me more likely to binge, but because of the massive restriction I'd practiced for so many months, it also made me feel very scared and anxious. Frankly, I'd become very afraid of food in general. Clearly, this madness had to end.

Ever since that realization, I've been feeling great. I am no longer trying to "fix" what's not broken and have embraced pleasure with food again; it's a very freeing, serene experience when you instinctively eat moderately and with healthy foods simply because you want to. I do have a deep respect for functional medicine. I admire and believe in its philosophy of peeling back the layers of malaise to get to the root cause and not simply prescribing medicine as a quick fix. I do not dispute for a moment that many millions of people suffer from very real and dangerous food allergies. These diagnoses need to be dealt with and handled in such a way as to make the patient feel empowered as to what they can eat to feel less deprived. On the flip side, it's important to remember that blood tests can be imperfect or marred or just plain wrong. Maybe I should have dug deeper; maybe I should have gone for a second opinion. I made a personal choice to stop being so frantic and to listen to my body instead, and to put my trust in my inner dietician. I intuitively felt that these particular test results were wrong and psychologically harmful for me as well.

As I sit here with my whole grain pasta with broccoli and freshly grated parmesan, I smile at the lovely meal waiting for me. I feel peace instead of fear and anticipation instead of shame. *And really, isn't this how it should be?*

HEALING COMES IN WAVES

My revelations surrounding my health and the cognitive dissonance I was experiencing in my career made me realize that I had an important message to share with others, and I felt it was time to tap into that. The tipping point came when I went to visit a friend in New York who had established a robust life coaching practice. I peppered her with questions about how she went about doing it and fantasized my entire train ride home about whether I had the skill and the wherewithal to attempt opening up my own practice. My hesitation was palpable because I had been so comfortable and secure in my job for so long yet felt an incredible itch to move onto whatever came next.

I started researching health coaching programs and thanks to the dizzying array of shiny objects to chase in the internet ether, I found my perfect program. It was the program that would change my life. It helped me heal and gave me the confidence I had been seeking to finally give up dieting once and for all, but better than that, it gave me the tools to help others do the same thing. I found The Institute for the Psychology of Eating. The program encompassed all of the things that I felt were lacking at my current job. I would become an Eating Psychology Coach and finally learn how to peel back the painful layers of denial, exposing the real reasons that so many of us spend our whole lives embracing an unsustainable dieting culture. It also addressed related issues such as poor digestion, chronic fatigue, and mind/body nutrition, etc. It was as if this program was tailor made for me and I jumped on the opportunity to enroll immediately.

GYMNASIA AND HEALING THROUGH MOVEMENT

Another fortuitous opportunity came my way during my research phase, which I'll now lovingly refer to as the "why Jenny is a weight gain machine and what to do about it" phase. I had always exercised, at least since the age of eighteen when, as you'll recall, I obstinately promised myself I would never, ever, ever resort to getting liposuction. I had accepted that I would never be a runner or star soccer player and I was at peace with that, but over time, I fell into an alternating routine of step aerobics, which I was shockingly adept at, even with the complicated step patterns and intense elliptical workouts (the elliptical was my frenemy) that lasted ninety minutes or more. Neither were particularly enjoyable, the latter only being tolerable while watching cooking shows on the Food Network to distract me (think of the irony there, readers).

I had read a lot about the benefits of yoga and also of lifting and swinging kettlebells, but the former felt a little too woo-woo for me and the latter seemed too intense. After all, my goal wasn't to become all bulky and overly muscular so what was the point, right? In addition, I had always loved to be in nature and went on really challenging hikes and walks, but I never considered that to be exercise. To me, exercise meant sweating in a gym for an hour or more and feeling insanely miserable the whole time. At the time, I had no concept of how much more exercising could be and how much joy it could bring me outside of decreasing my pant size.

I started with hot yoga. A neighbor and friend of mine strongly urged me to go with her one afternoon and my life was forever changed. I'll admit that I went in with a bad attitude and internally rolling my eyes at the "oms," "namastes," and Ujjayi breathwork. Despite my opposition, I was transformed when I realized just how difficult yoga is and how it forced me to come up against my edge of discomfort and just stand there and deal with it. It was a revelation. The temperature made me even more present, and after a few months of practicing this kind of yoga, I was completely hooked. My relationship with stress changed. My strongly negative reactions to the requisite annoyances in life, like kids fighting, traffic jams, and waiting in line, were mitigated thanks to yoga. I was embracing woo-woo and it was only the beginning!

Next, I began crowdsourcing on Facebook. It was time for a personal trainer as I had decided that I needed to build muscle to help raise my metabolic rate. Two people directed me to a little-known exercise studio called Gymnasia in West Newton, MA and specifically suggested I work with someone named Everett.

Gymnasia was a complete eye-opener for me. It was challenging, but its emphasis on good form, body weight focused movement, kettlebells, and sustainability was enticing and so different than anything I had ever experienced around movement before. I signed up for six one-on-one sessions with Everett. The very first thing I told him was that if he could help me lose weight, I'd give him my first-born. Losing weight was still front and center in my mind and now I was directing this squarely at the studio and Everett as a last ditch effort to help me. In the six weeks that followed, I learned how to hold a kettlebell. I re-learned how to do a summersault. I hung on gymnastic rings and swung like a monkey. I learned where my strength resided (my lower body) and increased my reps and weight steadily throughout my time there.

Everett taught me about how movement and play are intertwined and how each can be a source of both inner and outer strength to tap into when I felt swayed by the tumultuous tides of body angst and dieting. He taught me to dig in, to understand where my notions of dieting and body image came from, and how to consciously and respectfully create stop-gaps to ward against it. He encouraged me to use movement as a means for creating balance and sustainability and to parlay that strength into my everyday life. What had become a one-woman obsessive mission to lose weight slowly dissipated into excitement about what new tricks and feats my body could accomplish. Here's a letter I wrote to the team at Gymnasia and to Everett after four weeks of working out there:

Dear Josh, Jessica, Everett, and everyone at Gymnasia!

Just two days before starting privates with Everett at Gymnasia, I had a full body assessment done through a workplace initiative and was very disappointed with the results. Despite a very healthy vegan diet and tons of daily exercise, I have been unable to lose weight or see significant changes in my body. I've tried desperately for almost five years now, doing it on my own. This is especially challenging for me emotionally because I work at a weight and health management company and help others to lose weight and exercise more every day—so why couldn't I do it myself??

Anyway, I just had the assessment re-done after almost four weeks and I feel like the results are pretty amazing and wanted to share with you!

Visceral fat: went from 17-15 (under 10 to be healthy)
Muscle mass: went up .9 pounds!
BMI: dropped .6 points
Lost 3.2 pounds
Percent body fat: dropped 1.7 percent!!!

All in less than a month! I am literally floored by this. It's clear to me that while I lead a healthy and active life, I haven't been using my body in the most efficient way to burn calories or build muscle. I've been spinning my wheels, so to speak, and I feel like I'm on the cusp of a big change, and for that, I am so grateful!

I don't know what the next two months will bring with the sixty-day challenge but I am feeling very hopeful and positive about making these changes for the first time in five years. I can't wait for the rest of the challenge, and hopefully my journey at Gymnasia beyond that as well.

I told Everett when we had our first consult that I would give him my first-born child if he was able to enact any change in my body and help me lose weight. Well, I'm sorry to say that my daughter is about to leave for sleep-away camp, so alas, you will have to make do with a heartfelt THANK YOU!

Have a happy and healthy rest of the week.

Best regards,

Jenny Berk

You'll note that, despite some progress, I was still pretty data-driven and weight loss focused. That was soon to change.

Here's the conflicted place I was in just merely five months after I sent that letter:

Hi Everett,

I hope you're doing well! Have you finished Middlesex yet? Other books I highly recommend (other than Unbroken) are Infidel, 11/22/63 (long, but worth it) and Cutting for Stone. Amazing reads...

Anyway, I've really been in my head lately about the weighing in thing. This is the longest period of time in my life where I haven't gotten on the scale. There are some clear benefits of this but there are some other elements to weighing in that I haven't fully explored.

Pros of weighing in:

1. I get basic, important weekly feedback on how I am doing with respect to calories-in and calories-out, which guides me with my future decisions about how much I eat and how much I expend in exercise. Also, it can reinforce the good behaviors that I do daily.

2. I have days where I feel amazing in my skin and body, days where I don't care about the scale, and then days where I really don't feel good. It's those days where the clothes don't fit right that make me feel like I need to know if it's in my head or based on other things that I need to quickly address.

3. I feel bad because I am basically lying at work. Every staff member is part of a role modeling coaching loop there. As part of that, I have to report my food records, exercise, calories, and I have to give my weight each week to someone at our corporate office. For the last four weeks, I've been lying about it and I don't feel good about that. It also goes against some of the tenets of my company philosophy and what I ask my patients to do (weigh in weekly).

4. I have a yearly physical coming up in a few weeks and I know they are going to weigh me and I am terrified that if I don't weigh in first and get on the scale there, I am going to be very upset if it's not the number I'm expecting.

Cons for weighing in:

1. There are days I feel incredible and I don't need a scale to tell me otherwise.

2. In the last month, I have hurt my back and not exercised for a week and a half, went to NYC with a lot of unstructured eating and binged, ahem, I mean splurged on Halloween, and I am so scared to see if that has affected the scale negatively.

There are definitely other measures for health and wellness. I know that to be true, honestly, I do. But, to be frank, I am scared that if I'm not constantly vigilant, I could gain an incredible amount of weight despite the wonderful healthy behaviors I engage in daily. It's fear of the unknown. It's quite the dichotomy—feeling in control and completely out of control at the same time.

Would you be willing to talk through some of this with me on Wednesday? I'd really appreciate it. You don't need to reply to this email. We can just talk then. I just wanted to get my thoughts down for you.

Thank you so much Everett!! Have a wonderful weekend!

Jenny

By the end of my first year at Gymnasia, my tune had completely changed. I had stopped focusing on the number on the scale for good and started caring more about the very behaviors that felt so intrinsic to me all along to be healthy. A remarkably positive change within me was afoot.

April 14th, 2015

Dear Everett,

It's been almost a year since I first walked into Gymnasia and met you. I started this journey by crowdsourcing on Facebook, asking if anyone knew of a really good trainer/gym that I could try as an alternative to Boston Sports Club, which was, after five years, making me uninspired and weary. Thank goodness to Sallie who responded and helped shepherd me to you guys.

When I first joined, my main and singular objective, as you know, was to lose weight. In fact, you probably remember that I had a certain goal of losing seven to ten pounds in two months to use as an empirical metric to determine if I was being "successful" with this new endeavor.

If you had asked me a year ago whether weight loss would end up being a tertiary goal for me, I would have both laughed in your face and been angered by even the notion.

I have grown and changed in ways I can't even describe through this process. Could I actually live in a world where strength trumps weight loss? Where ability supplants dress size? It appears I am. I have been dieting and struggling my whole life to lose weight, to the point of obsession. Never would it have occurred to me that there could be a deep and lasting satisfaction from the process of getting strong and moving my body in amazing ways. Never would I have imagined that I could be more fierce and strong and confident than I was in my twenties. Never would I have expected that I could feel beautiful even at my heaviest weight ever and at this age.

This, in large part, is due to you, Everett. I'm not going to lie. There will always be a part of me that wants to lose weight, but it, indeed, has become a secondary goal for me. I am both excited and motivated by tackling my next challenge, my next feat, and my next kettlebell color. I garner immense gratification doing all of these things—all with you at the helm, supporting and inspiring me every step of the way.

This inner/outer strength I now have at the core has emanated to all other parts of my life, from pondering a career change to wearing a bikini again, it's all due, in part, to this process and to you and Gymnasia. I will always be grateful for what you guys have brought to my life.

This is what my arms looked like about a year ago, after attempting to do a forward roll. Remember how deflated and embarrassed I felt? Last week at play day, I was rolling all over the place with a buoyancy and ease that felt like I was frolicking! A year ago, I could not even handle and grip the kettlebell, let alone swing 24kg. I could not do any kind of inversion at all, let alone a headstand.

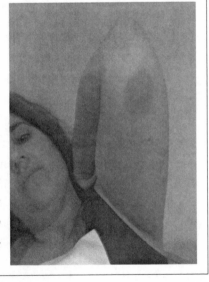

From bruises to blossoming athlete:

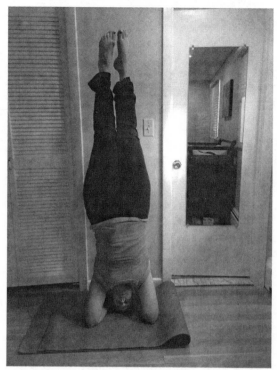

Doing a headstand for the first time in my life.

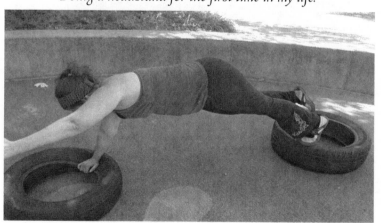

Playing with tires!

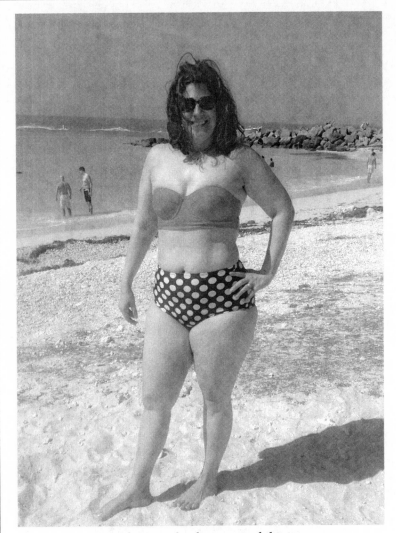

No longer afraid to wear a bikini!

With gratitude and admiration,

Jenny

This complete transformation in my relationship with exercise left me feeling free. I felt joyful, and quite frankly, I felt unstoppable. Along with the Institute for the Psychology of Eating, I credit Gymnasia, specifically Everett, and this type of movement path for freeing me from my dieting shackles and helping me to find the courage to finally leave my job and pursue my true passion.

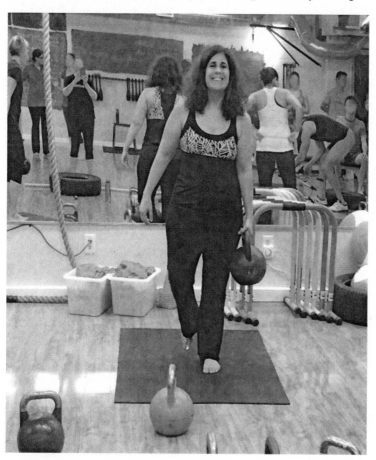

I finally understand what loving exercise is all about and it's very freeing. I'm not saying everyone would find the same satisfaction in this type of exercise that I've chosen to do, but I do know this: Humans were meant to be active and everyone has the ability to find something active that moves their heart and soul just as much as their bodies. Might that be dancing? Hiking? Zumba? Prancercising? It really doesn't matter.

Just go out and find it! Your heart AND your body will thank you.

BOUDOIR OR BUST

I have an amazing friend, Abby, the figurative nude photographer, with whom I feel a kindred spirit with and an abundance of trust. She is also the survivor of an eating disorder. Abby is one of my closest confidants and has always been someone who I am able to express and share my process with in real time as triumphs and setbacks occurred for me. I had always been aware of her amazing talent and craft by the beautiful nudes embossed on metal frames that adorn her home. Abby's use of light and shadow is a marvel to me and exquisitely captures the incredible nuances and beauty of the human body. Her focus on body diversity and interest in shooting people of all ages and shapes is even more alluring to me. It is part of what makes her work so fascinating. After a heart-to-heart we shared one evening over dinner, Abby suggested, or rather insisted, that she photograph me. I was intrigued and terrified at first, but after some thought, I decided this was something I ought to do to help heal myself from years of my own body shaming and insecurity. The experience was nothing short of exhilarating.

I trust Abby unconditionally, so being naked in front of her was a hurdle that wasn't too difficult. What was harder was becoming comfortable in my own skin, moving and posing naturally without trying to impress anyone. Abby's first comment to me was that I had a fine "padunkadunk," and that instantly made me laugh, which helped put me at ease.

After two hours in her studio, I felt gloriously bold, alive, and sexy. In fact, I actually felt effervescent. Despite being apprehensive about seeing the photos when they were done, it did, in fact, have a healing effect on me. I was proud that I stepped way out of my comfort zone and challenged myself emotionally. I was very pleased with the photos and grateful that she was able to create images that I wholeheartedly adored. It would become one of the last rungs in my healing process.

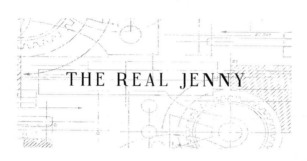

THE REAL JENNY

I was steadily starting to heal both my relationship with food and exercise, and also finally showing my body a little kindness and compassion. I started to fully respect everything it has done for me and all the amazing ways I get to show up in the world because of the body I have. I started to practice gratitude for my body—my uterus for having the ability to birth three amazing, healthy children, my legs for allowing me to walk on glorious beaches, and my arms for their ability to hold and hug the ones I love. I morphed from body loathing to full respect and kindness, and guess what? My body responded kindly. It had been waiting all these years for me to finally raise the white flag, to show it some love, and to stop punishing it into a weight it clearly didn't want to be. It was the most freeing and peaceful experience I had ever had. I said goodbye to restrictive dieting for good and I haven't looked back.

WHY I'LL NEVER SAY THESE FOUR WORDS AGAIN

"Do I look fat?"

Come on, we've all asked this of someone—a spouse, a friend, a clothing store salesperson. We say it with hope, with longing, and with some concern as well. We think that, somehow, whatever reply comes from the lips of these individuals will relieve us of our body image stress. This loaded question not only puts a lot of pressure on the person you're asking, but it also strips you of your own power.

How does it strip you of your power? Simply because if you turn to others to determine your beauty, it shrouds your own ability to view yourself as such. In some ways, it is even passing the buck. It is putting onto someone else your own negative body image anxiety.

Perception is a funny thing. As human beings, perception plays an enormous role in how we view the world. Is the glass half empty or is it half full? Perception. Was that dress white and gold or blue and black? Perception. "Do I look fat?" It is just one person's perception of reality that may be completely different than someone else's. What is important is your own perception of self. This is what most of us need to work on most of all. We need to stop trying to impress everyone else. The truth is that when we accept ourselves and project confidence, grace, and comfort in our skin, that is when other people notice anyway!

If a scale says I'm overweight but I actually feel thin and beautiful, which is the reality? If my BMI says I'm at a "normal" weight, but I feel bloated and disgusting and huge, again, which is the reality?

Our perceptions are fickle. There are times I actually feel like I am twenty-five years old, when I think I look as though I weigh 115 pounds. And other times, I just feel or perceive myself to be dumpy and looking much older than I am. My theory is that when we ask others whether or not we look good, look fat, or anything else related to appearance, we are actually trying to reconcile some incongruent perception of ourselves in that moment; to make other people either confirm or deny our own experience of self!

How about trying this next time you feel compelled to ask other people's opinion about how you look? Stop for a minute and close your eyes. Take some deep breaths and try to sit with the uncomfortable feelings that are coming up for you in that moment. Where is the anxiety stemming from? Is it possible you're in a bad mood about something else? Is it possible that something you ate made you feel different or uncomfortable in your skin? Did something happen to challenge your sense of self, like a benign comment from a coworker that you perceived as a slight? Because we have this gift of perception, we also have this ability to choose to believe and assume the best in any situation as well. When we can stop, breathe, and tolerate the uncomfortable feelings that are coming up in the moments just before giving away our power to someone else, we have an opportunity to reclaim our power. We have the ability to believe nothing other than that we are beautiful, ageless souls. It's all up to the individual.

Because, after all, from my perspective, there is only one answer to the question, "Do I look fat?" and it is this: "To me, you look like you, like who you are supposed to be right now, and to me, this is beautiful. This is enough."

It was at this point in my journey that I finally felt equipped with the courage and strength to find my own voice and philosophy, and to share what I had been experiencing with the rest of the world. In fact, I felt driven to give the gifts that I had found through my training and my realignment with exercise with as many other people as I could. I knew it was time to leave my job.

I'm now living my dreams. I lead a healthy, balanced, diet-free life with plenty of movement, yummy plant-based food, and meditation. I have an abundance of energy to give to myself and to the ones I love now that I no longer obsess about my body weight and about every bite of food I eat. I trust myself and I no longer feel called to overeat, binge eat, or emotionally eat because I place no restrictions on myself. When there were so many rules and restrictions, it led to almost a constant desire to break those rules and do it excessively. I have dessert whenever I want, but I find I want it far less frequently—another amazing by-product of no longer denying myself after so many years. We all deserve to experience pleasure with food. Human beings are biologically wired to seek pleasure and avoid pain so why is it that we have such moral objections to seeking pleasure in food? Why is it that words like "disgusting" and "over-indulgent" are associated with the sensuality and enjoyment around food?

My healing gave me the courage to help other people by no longer confirming or accepting these societal norms that beauty shows up only in one way. I actively challenge the notion that there is one cookie cutter diet right for every person and, instead,

I promote discovering one's own trust in body wisdom, for only you know what is right for your own body.

DIETARY DETECTIVE

If you're like me, in my adult life, I have followed many diets, food trends, and "experts" who have told me what to eat, when to eat, and how much of it to eat. If there were a gimmicky juice cleanse that claimed to increase metabolism or a paleo for vegans diet that I hadn't tried yet, I'd be all over it.

That was then.

That was before I realized that only I am an expert when it comes to what is good for my own body. While I greatly respect physicians, dieticians and nutritionists who know how different foods affect the body and can roughly determine for people what macro and micronutrients we each should have to be healthy and fully nourished, I have realized that most prescribed "diets" are just a simple tweaking of the basic fat/protein/carb trio in one fashion or another. Low carb, low fat. Low this, high that. Eat this, don't eat that. It's enough to drive anyone crazy!

I have learned that each person has bio-individuality (the concept that no one diet works for every person all the time) and each of us needs to respect our own special nature regarding food. We need to listen more to our own inner experts rather than relying on the wisdom of others. It's dangerous to say that there is one perfect diet that everyone should follow. You may find that, at some points in your life, you need specific types of diets—a cleansing or detoxifying diet when you've indulged a lot during the holidays, an optimizing diet, say, if you're training for a marathon. For some, spicy food is beneficial. For others, it creates GERD. For some, dairy is queen, and for others, it causes major digestive issues. You have different needs when you're pregnant and when you go through menopause, when you exercise and when you don't exercise, when you're getting over a cold and when you are getting over a stomach bug. How can anyone claim to say they have the diet that is best for you, bar none, without knowing the minutia of each individual person at any particular moment? You're the expert here!

From an evolutionary perspective, it's absolutely absurd that we would fathom taking whole food groups out of our diet, as in low-carb diets or even some paleo inspired diets. Can you imagine asking a lion to take out antelope and stick to the leaner zebra for thirty days for optimal health?! How and when have we stopped trusting our own intuition about what our bodies need to be healthy? Is it simply the abundance of choices we have available to us? Or is it perhaps the fact that healthy, organic food from the earth and from healthy animals is less available and oftentimes more expensive? Maybe we are so stressed and busy that we just want to outsource our eating habits to someone else. That makes sense, but it also compounds my belief that we have completely lost touch with inner wisdom. Our bodies are always talking to us. We have just ceased to listen!

We have so many food decisions to make each day. Brian Wansink, of the book *Mindless Eating*, suggests that Americans make up to 200 food related decisions a day. That is a lot of decisions! Freedom of choice is both a luxury and a curse. We are a choice-loving people, but research also shows we develop decision fatigue easily, and when that decision quota is up, we quickly become overwhelmed and make decisions based on what's easiest (i.e. fast food, processed foods etc.).

Another problem that prevents us from being able to tune into inner wisdom is the fact that we are literally addicted to food. How can we possibly make sound food judgments when the chemicals in our favorite processed foods keep us in a vicious cycle of binge/restrict, binge/restrict? We know these foods are "bad" for us, yet because it's a socially acceptable indulgence and widely available, we often end up eating it anyway. When we eat it, the reward centers in our brains light up, releasing dopamine, which activates the cues for wanting more and more and more of it. So, what do we do? We go cold turkey, which works only for a short time until we lose our willpower, binge on said food, and begin the cycle yet again.

So, what is the solution to all of this?

Become your own dietary detective.

Learn to slow down when you eat and when you make decisions about eating. Practice mindful eating. See how your body feels and responds to certain foods. What makes you feel nourished? What foods give you energy? Which make you feel fatigued? You are your own expert when it comes to your diet. You no longer need to rely only on the "experts" and diet authors, but on your own blueprint from within. Once you learn the basics of slowing down, tuning in and experimenting, something magical happens. You instinctively know what and when and how much to eat, just like the lion does. There is peace and freedom from this place, taking you away from all the clutter of food trends, dietary hype, and government sponsored suggested plates. Yes, it takes time. Yes, it takes practice, and yes, you may need support. The end result is you trusting yourself for the needs of your body, and that's a pretty phenomenal achievement.

For the past two years, I have been sharing my passion and commitment to a mindful and empowering relationship between food and body with other women, men, and adolescents. I have created online courses and signature talks that have helped people in immeasurable ways. In my work, I constantly emphasize how important it is that we lift the veil and confront the detrimental societal ideals we have in place regarding what constitutes health and beauty. We need to get our hands dirty and talk to our children openly and honestly about these tough topics that will inevitably affect them. This is so that when the time comes, they already have tools in place to help them navigate toward their truth. It took me a long time to peel back the thick layers of body-loathing, but I kept pushing forward, and eventually, I found vulnerability and beauty where I once knew only disappointment. I want that for every person, including you, so that you, too, can shed the shackles of body-shame and the hate that keeps you restricted from sharing your vast and amazing gifts with the world.

I was a boring, narrow minded person when I was a chronic dieter. I had nothing really interesting to discuss unless you wanted to talk about calorie intake vs. output. Now, I'm exploring all facets of who I am and I'm learning so much more about what lights me up, where my skills reside, and how I can contribute to the world in a more meaningful way. Some people may wonder if I miss being thinner and the answer is a resounding, "Of course!" Please know that in an ideal world I would love nothing more than to easily maintain a lower body weight, but I have accepted that this is not what my body wants for me. Sure, I could put in the heroic efforts I once did until I reached my goals, but for what? I am so incredibly happy and at peace. Why on Earth would I want to go back to that rigid way of life? Despite being a higher weight, I am healthy and active. I eat nutritious food and feel amazing in my skin. What's not to love? No scale or BMI chart can tell me differently.

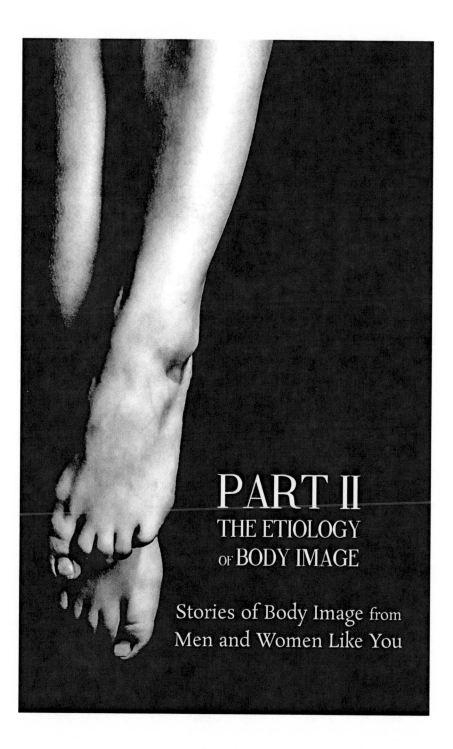

PART II
THE ETIOLOGY
of BODY IMAGE

Stories of Body Image from
Men and Women Like You

"Most of us spend our lives protecting ourselves from losses that have already happened."

—GENEEN ROTH

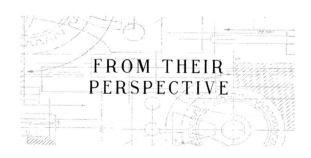

FROM THEIR
PERSPECTIVE

I f you think that my story is unique, I'll be the first to tell you
that that is anything but the truth. In my research and countless interviews with men and women all over the country, I
found strikingly similar patterns in the origins of how people
come to shape their identity with their body image. It is often
fraught with pain, shame, hatred and discomfort, both physically and emotionally. I sought to better understand whether one's
body image is determined externally, let's say from parental sources, peers or media, or whether it was coming strictly from within.

We are the only species on Earth that even has the ability to
hate or criticize its physical form. Last I checked, I didn't see my
cat primping in front of the mirror or restricting her kitty chow.
I happily acknowledge that there are some individuals that grew
up with a healthy sense of self and body image, and some who
only struggled later in life, if at all. Unfortunately, those were the
minority of people I interviewed.

In this next section, you will hear from these body image
warriors. You'll get an honest look into what many people experienced as children and into adulthood and how the sense of

self can change over the years. The men and women interviewed range in age from twenty-two all the way to seventy. In this section, it is explored when one first noticed they have an opinion of their body, what measures, if any, they have taken to change their exterior, and much more.

It was a revelation to learn about these journeys and to know that this is a sad and systemic problem human beings face. While brainstorming about the questions I would ask all of these gracious and brave interviewees, the first topic that piqued my interest was physical self-awareness. My hypothesis going into the research was that this probably occurred at a very young age, definitely by elementary school, but maybe even as early as four or five years old. I was surprised to learn that, for some, these opinions didn't become clear or evident until adolescence or even well into adulthood.

QUESTION: *When was the first time you noticed you had an opinion of your body? What was that opinion and how old were you?*

"When I was twelve years old, wearing a bikini and my ribs stuck out."
-Heidi W., 44

"When I was fourteen and I had just given birth to my daughter, my mother told me that because of all of my stretch marks, no man would ever want me."
-Nikki B., 51

"I was very small as a child and was very aware because people always told me—it didn't really bother me then—I capitalized on being "cute," but in adolescence, it all changed and I was aware that nothing was right."
-Emily S., 62

"I think high school. I remember seeing a photo of my younger self and thinking, 'Holy smokes. I look like alien!' I was a VERY skinny kid and apparently had a big head!"
-Monique N., 32

"As an eight-year-old, when I was put on my first diet at summer camp."
-Cathy B., 66

"Super young. Maybe even four years old! My mom told me that every time I went to get my hair cut, I said I wanted a straight haircut, meaning, I wanted to get my frizzy, curly, messy hair straightened at age four. I already had an opinion that straight hair was prettier than my curly hair."
-Talia K., 24

"Probably when I was around thirty years old."
-Melissa M., 52

"At ten, when I first got my period."
-AFS, 38

"From about three years old, I was aware that I was chubby and larger than other kids."
-Joe B., 35

"About seventeen, I felt I had a large middle. However, when I think back to it, I was quite normal. I just didn't know it then."

-Lisa F., 66

Body image was not specifically related to size, as you can see from these answers. It also pertained to curliness of hair, stretch marks, head size, and more. Fears or insecurities about being too skinny or small or short were just as prevalent as being large or fat. While my story is only from the perspective of feeling and being larger than the other girls my age, I discovered the pain, awkwardness, and self-consciousness that so many of us feel about all aspects of our bodies.

One of the things I wonder about to this day is the degree of influence on internal versus external self-perception. In other words, do we develop opinions about the acceptability or beauty of our bodies based on our own voices, or do we gradually develop these ideas based on comments or values placed on us from other people, like our parents, our peers, or society? One of the arcs in my own story was this constant dichotomy and internal struggle over conforming to perceived norms of thinness and actively defying it, knowing deep down that I was just fine the way I was. I now believe that while my own voice was telling me I was fine the way I am, I was ultimately unable to keep that aloft against the tides of other people's harsh opinions and judgments, which kept me in fear and unable to listen to my own wisdom. In the next interview question, I sought to understand if others also fell prey to outside or external opinions about their appearance based on their own opinions.

QUESTION: *Do you remember an incident or experience where someone made a comment about your appearance that had a lasting impression on you? Be specific.*

"Yes, I remember in college (although, I do remember the guy specifically) that I was told to my face by a guy that I had a radio face (the kind of face that's not pretty enough for a camera). I also remember around fourteen years of age, being told by my mother, prior to a dinner event with family and guests, to 'fix my face,' meaning to go put makeup on so that I would look presentable."
-Cydney P., 37

"My dad was always on me about my weight, even when I wasn't really fat. And my mom, instead of backing me up, would say, "Oh, you have such a nice figure, if you'd just lose weight..."
-Susan A., 42

"After giving birth to my daughter, my hormones ran wild. I began having cystic acne on my face and was faced with public humiliation everywhere. Small children, though innocent, always seemed to find me in a room full of friends or just at the grocery store and ask me what was wrong with my face. All eyes would then turn to me and everything went quiet around me. How do I answer this without crying?"
-Catie M., 31

"When I was twelve, I lost twenty-five pounds, and all of a sudden, grown-ups were offering me dessert and saying things like, 'You deserve it.' It stayed with me—the idea that fatter people don't deserve dessert, but if you are thin, you do."
-Tami W., 40

"My boyfriend, when I was fourteen, called me 'chubby' and it was the first time it occurred to me that I might not have a good body. I think the choice of going on a diet was somehow not as connected to feeling like my body wasn't good enough as this experience was."
-Carly M., 39

"Yes, I remember coming home from college after being away most of my freshman year in Boston, and an old family friend commenting on how good I looked. She asked what I had done, and I wasn't sure how to answer her. All I could think of was that I smoked a pack of cigarettes per day, drank a ton of coffee, hardly slept, and had lost seventeen pounds in that first year of college."
-AFS, 38

"My best friend told me at age twelve that if I didn't stop eating and get thinner that she didn't want to be around me. I remember being so afraid of losing her."
-Kirsten P., 40

"I liked a popular, cute boy around fourth grade. He and I were friends, but I had a major crush on him. He told our mutual friends that if I went to diet camp over the summer and lost weight that he would be my boyfriend. Funny thing is, he even offered to pay for this diet camp. He really wanted a girlfriend who was not fat."
-Kelly R., 51

"My grandparents on my father's side made a comment about my chubby cheeks. I was not very close to them and only saw them once in a while. I remember thinking, *How can people who are supposed to love you make an awful comment like that?*"
-Caren C., 56

"Boys always commented on my feet—wearing boats or skis for shoes. I would hide my feet by sitting Indian style or curl them up under my desk. I started slouching a lot after a family photographer complained about my height because it affected how his picture looked."
-Dayna S., 36

"There were many. In elementary school, people used to comment on my weight and how much I liked to eat. At the age of eleven, I decided to stop eating to lose weight. I became very active and very restrictive of my food for the next almost twenty years. In high school, even though I barely ate and worked out hours a day, people still commented that I had a "fat ass" or something along those lines. For years, I felt of less value physically than many fit and pretty girls. One of the many issues with this was that I was 115 pounds and 5'4". As women and little girls, we are instilled with a belief that we need to look a certain way to be of more value and that is how I led my life for years."
-Cherri J., 34

"I remember being told that at about two years old my pediatrician told my parents he wanted to be my agent when I played in the NFL. I experienced a lot of mixed emotions growing up. As a boy, bigger is better, so in some ways, I was proud of being bigger. However, I was teased, singled out, and picked on by kids, teachers, coaches, friends, parents, etc., so I knew I wasn't big in the 'right way.'"
-Joe B., 35

"I don't. I do remember my mother ALWAYS being on a diet or talking about diet and exercise and weight, and I remember cutting lots of clippings out of newspapers about how to have a flat stomach, what foods to eat, what exercises to do to stay thin."
-Julie K., 41

"Yes! At age fifteen, my parents pretty much told me I was chunky (I wasn't) and then sent me to a personal trainer because I was too young to sign up for a gym membership. I remember being open to it, but I didn't really want to. From a young age, I always participated in some kind of sport, like gymnastics, dance, soccer, softball and track. At that age, my interests shifted from sports to photography and I think my parents were worried I'd get out of shape. Then, from age seventeen and on, I was a total gym nut and still am. I can't lie. I enjoy the effects from working out (visually) on my body. But my main motivations for working out now are fitting into my clothes, staying flexible, and maintaining my core and leg strength for snowboarding, which is my favorite sport.

Another instance, at age eighteen, my mom used to make comments on what I was eating: 'You're having another doughnut?' 'You're having another slice of pizza?' She's very thin and health conscious. When I was in college, we did several detox/cleanses together. Of course, the effects never lasted!"
-Talia K., 24

The comments that had lasting impressions on people came from many sources—brothers, moms, dads, pediatricians, gym teachers, friends, strangers. It left me wondering, does the inner bully develop mostly because of constant body-shaming and bullying from others? Do we internalize their comments and slowly accept them as gospel? Are we unable to unfetter ourselves from outside perceptions, thus distorting our own reality? The amazing, flowy sundress you thought you looked so good in when you were leaving the house suddenly makes you feel frumpy when you pass by the first reflection in a window or later on in a photo your friend sends of the two of you. But why?

WINDOW REFLECTIONS

To the young woman checking herself out in the window at that restaurant today: I see you pushing in your tummy, with a furtive sideways glance, critically judging yourself. I want to remind you that you are beautiful, you always have been, you always will be. You don't know it; you don't even see it. It causes me pain to see you harshly judging yourself without even uttering a word. It's painful because I know the feeling. I, too, had become intimately acquainted with every window or mirror reflection on every street corner. One window offers a rosy, thin reflection, while the very next one becomes shockingly unappealing. How is that even possible? It's the same person, same reflection, yet two vastly different experiences of self.

I see what you are doing—pretending to look inside the window and into the restaurant, trying not to appear vain. But really, you're seeing yourself; pushing, pulling, straightening your skirt, and hoping that by pulling it down at just the correct angle you will cover that part of your body you are insecure about today.

I see you quickly change emotional gears as your friend walks up to greet you. I wonder, though, if the painful feelings linger. Maybe you're thinking about how you look compared to your friend. Maybe, inside, you are planning your next diet while happily chatting away and catching up. Maybe you are anxiously thinking about how you didn't work out today yet. Maybe you are deciding to opt out of the yummy meal you were looking forward to for a Diet Coke instead.

To this woman I saw today and so many others, I see you. I hear you. I am you. I understand. There is freedom from this tortuous path. Even though it's challenging and it takes time, you can have a better relationship with your body and with food. It can be done in a way you never would have thought to pursue before, by going towards the pain rather than away. Be mindful rather than mindlessly numbing out. Love your way into a better relationship with food rather than simply having a black and white, "good" food, "bad" food attitude. I've crawled my way out of these food and body shackles over the last two years and there is a tremendous amount of peace and freedom in that.

Let's get you there too.

Throughout my life, even at the nadir of my body-loathing, there were parts of my body that I really enjoyed. My hair, for instance, was enviably thick, long, and shiny. I loved the compliments and the attention so much that I let just about anyone run their fingers through it. One boy in my English class did just that. Every week, he would sit behind me and use my hair as his own personal comfort blanket, curling strands around his fingers then letting them go again. Hair, or lack thereof, plays a very important role in our identity and self-worth. No matter what my size was, my hair was always my trusty, consistently beautiful companion. My booty, though, was the part of my body I was most self-conscious about. I wanted to know if others were able to isolate a part of their body that they had always been truly able to appreciate and love.

Conversely, I was curious to find out if all men and women have a particular part of their bodies that took the brunt of all their negative self-talk and body loathing, and if so, why? That we can have such revulsion for our backsides, for instance, yet be kind about our lips, hair or eyes, amazes me. Where do these subjective opinions come from? The answers were so varied and remarkable. Some people admitted they loved themselves unconditionally or that they loved their heart. For others, it was the opposite with some finding it hard to find a single aspect of their bodies that they loved and appreciated.

QUESTION: *What is one part of your body that you love?* For the record, 5.7% of all respondents loved their legs, 3.8% loved their bellies, and 3.8% loved their hearts!

"All of it!"
-Charlotte N., 43

"My heart."
-Nikki B., 51

"Eyes, brain."
-Anonymous

"My hair. It's long and wavy and thick and it reminds me of mermaid hair."
-Sarah M., 24

"My breasts."
-AFS, 38

"It used to be my eyes, but now they just look tired."
-Lisa P., 36

"Love is a strong word, but my nose is pretty good! I like my eyes too."
-Emily S. 63

"I always thought I had nice hands. In fact, sometimes, people say I should be a hand model because my nails are perfectly shaped!"
-Marie P., 40

"I love my shape. There are so many things."
-Cheri J., 34

"My belly because it carried my daughter."
-Carly M., 39

On the opposite side of the spectrum, there was no dearth of body parts that my interviewees despised about themselves. Breasts were a source of discomfort for many I interviewed. Some viewed theirs as too big and some as too small! Who, in fact, actually determined the "goldilocks" version of boobies??

QUESTION: *What is one part of your body that you dislike or are uncomfortable with?*

"My hair is broken in a lot of places from being pregnant and it makes me feel self-conscious."
-Carly M., 39

"Can I only choose one? I guess I would have to say my thighs. "I hate the way they look in a bathing suit."
-Heidi W., 44

"OY! Stomach and thighs. Oh, and don't forget the flabby arms."
-Emily S., 63

"My backside. I did a health program a year ago where I had to take a photo before and after the program of my front, side, and

back. I could not believe the photo of my backside was actually ME. It was COVERED with cellulite. I kind of ignore it now. I also have hunched shoulders."
-Lisa P., 36

"I don't like the way any of my body looks physically. My weight is a big issue, but again, I still don't really like my face."
-Anita T., 51

"Can I say all? Really, from the neck down, I'd change something about every part of me if I could. Right now, it's really my upper arms. I do exercise and strength training, but I still have that upper arm jiggle. (I think ladies will know what I mean.)"
-Anonymous

"Hips have always been a struggle, and my belly continues to be a part that is asking for more love."
-Cydney P., 37

"My teeth. I have quite a crooked smile and I've never had braces or any correction to them. Most of the time, I don't even notice, but when I see myself on video, it really affects me. Not so much photos, but video. I think it makes me look like a young child."
-Monique N., 32

"When I stop working out for a week, my butt starts to get 'out of control,' as my mom would say. Also, my breasts have drooped significantly in my twenties, which is really, really sad. I don't like them at all!"
-Talia K., 24

"Mostly all of my body. I have struggled with disordered eating for seventeen years, and I still am not at peace with accepting my body for what it is."
-Jade B., 30

"Breasts (too small)!"
-Anonymous

"My breasts. They are much too big."
-Anonymous

And happily, there were a few people who genuinely loved and respected their bodies, imperfections and all.

"For the most part, I love my whole body these days. If I'm on my period, I retain quite a bit of water and will find myself feeling "thick" in my thighs. But I replace that with loving thoughts now!"
-Lauren S., 28

"I generally don't have trouble with any body part, but if I were pushed to give one, I would say tummy."
-Charlotte N., 43

"I'm generally pretty comfortable, but if I had to say, I think my stomach is the area that could use the most attention and is the first to go if I haven't been working out. Having just had a baby a few weeks ago, I hate how it looks right now, but I try not to count that. And since this is my second baby, I am optimistic about being able to get back into shape. I was able to get back to feeling good about my body after the first baby."
-Sara T., 31

> "At this point, I feel comfortable in my skin about 98% of the time. I especially love how I feel and look in well-fitting dress clothes. I also feel very comfortable in my skin during sex or just lounging around nude with my girlfriend."
> -Joe B., 35

Clearly, the people who are loving and accepting of themselves as-is are diminishing under the pressure to conform to some random and subjective ideal of beauty. Don't get me wrong. I do not judge those who want to make changes to their appearance. If it is something that is safe and will make that person feel amazing in their skin, then I say go for it. What concerns me is whether it's that person's own voice telling them to change or the voices of perfectionism and peer pressure speaking for them. I work with people to listen to and understand whose voice is speaking when they feel they want to make extreme changes.

When I asked my participants in what ways they had tried to change their exterior appearance in the past, the answers ran the gamut, ranging from bra stuffing all the way to surgical procedures like liposuction.

QUESTION: *Do you remember a time when you tried to change your exterior appearance? What measures did you take?*

"I stuffed my bra from fifth to ninth grade."
-Naomi R., 70

"Oh, yes. As a teenager, I did all sorts of diets and calorie restriction and over-exercising to try and slim down—South Beach Diet, Cabbage Soup Diet, running six miles every night, portion control, etc."
-Lauren S., 28

"I have had over $20k in cosmetic surgery in the past 3.5 years. "
-Nikki B., 51

"Yes. I have taken almost every measure with the exception of surgery. "
-Cherri J., 34

"I have dieted. I have had liposuction."
-Kelly R., 51

"I remember, in high school, I used to jog in place while watching General Hospital after school to try to lose weight. I have dieted and exercised to lose weight many times since. I have also dyed my hair from brown to blonde and red."
-Julie K., 41

"Many times. The most drastic is getting liposuction on my thighs in college. I convinced my dad to let me and that I'd pay him back. He didn't want to but, ultimately, let me. It was so deeply important to me at the time. Now, I look back and I feel sad for myself at that time, that I thought my self-worth and ability to be accepted and loved, mostly by a man, was connected to the ways my thighs looked."
-Anonymous

"I went to Overeaters Anonymous for over twenty years. I lost 100 pounds, and then started struggling. I now reject the program, finding it too judgmental and black/white thinking. After losing weight, I had breast reduction & a tummy tuck. These things have given me so much good feeling about myself."
-Alex F., 55

"I intentionally developed bulimia to lose weight. I didn't just accidentally stumble into bingeing and purging for I learned it from my mother. The funny thing is, she didn't raise me so I have no idea how I acquired her bad habits. When my parents were still together, I remember seeing my mother run out of the house to purge and hiding Tupperware containers of vomit in random places. My mother had and still has bulimia. As a child, I was appalled at the idea of throwing up. I cried every time it happened when I was sick. So how does one go

from hating it to, dare I say, "enjoying" it? I have no idea. I am not a doctor. I decided that I was going to lose weight, so I thought throwing up was a fast, easy solution that required little effort. Along with bulimia, I starved myself and over-exercised. The positive reinforcement of how I looked made me feel incredible. It was like adding fuel to the fire. I even did a bit of modeling, which was a dream of mine when I was younger. Who would stop something deemed "unhealthy" if your whole world thinks you are on fire? (My world. Not the world itself. I'm not a celebrity for God sake.) I never had as many compliments about my appearance as I did when I was sick."

-Jade B., 30

"Yes, I starved myself by eating only ice because that's what the girls in junior high told me."
-Kirsten P., 40

"I went through a twenty-year period wherein I would let my hair grow really long and then cut it all off—short, cropped. The change in identity that I could achieve by this one act was so fascinating to me."

-AFS, 38

"Ha! So many slimming methods and diets. Pretty much all of them, including wrapping myself in Saran wrap and extreme dieting methods that caused my hair to fall out."

-Deana M., 57

I was curious also to learn if men and women felt that a positive body image solely had to do with their size and their weight or if other factors were in play. With forty-eight participants answering this question, here is the breakdown of responses:

Do you believe that positive body image is weight dependent? (48 responses)

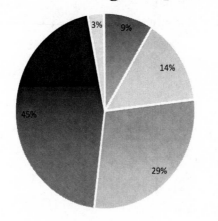

Yes, absolutely. I only feel good about myself when I weigh a certain amount. (9%)

No. (14%)

No, but it plays a role in addition to other factors. (29%)

Yes, but I also feel good when I practice other self-care measures. (45%)

Other (3%)

It was heartening to me that while most (45%) felt that body image is, indeed, weight dependent, that other important self-care measures like meditation, exercise, yoga, and eating a balanced diet made a difference.

Next, I sought to find out when, if at all, do people feel most comfortable and happy in their skin? Certainly, there had to be commonalities and patterns that emerge that point to ways to appreciate our "space suits" and love the skin we're in. Again, the answers presented a range of interesting ways people felt most comfortable. I was struck by how many participants felt most comfortable in their bodies when they were either engaging in an activity or hobby that they loved to do and felt authentic while doing it.

QUESTION: *Can you describe when you feel most comfortable in your skin (certain clothing, during sex, while running, etc.)?*

"I feel most comfortable when I'm at the barn riding horses, when I'm practicing belly dancing, and when I wear loose-fitting tops that are also low enough to reveal a little skin (or a lot)."
-Sarah M., 24

Many felt great when they were eating foods that felt nourishing and kind to their bodies.

"When I am nourishing my whole self with foods that have love and life in them, when I am working out and meditating daily, and when my husband comes in and says, 'Hello, beautiful.'"
-Nikki B., 51

"When I am eating mindfully, eating most of my meals at home, and getting in exercise I enjoy each day."
-Lauren S., 28

"When I've been eating in a healthful way."
-Lisa F., 66

Another common theme was comfort in their skin when doing certain exercises like yoga and running:

"Snowboarding for sure, running, and when I dress up for a nice event. I feel great when I actually put time into my appearance, but I don't have the time (or reason) to put on makeup every day."
-Talia K., 24

"I feel best when I am exercising. Just last night, I went to an awesome class that was super tough physically and I amazed myself that I was as strong and fit as I was. I was keeping up with extreme athletes and I was so proud! Non-size-six girls can kick butt too!"
-Erika S., 42

"During sex and yoga."
-AFS, 38

"Dancing!"
-Charlotte N., 43

"While at my barre class."
-Anonymous

Some felt confident when choosing to do acts of self-care, like meditation, dressing up, or getting a massage.

"When I have gone to extra effort with makeup, hair, and a coordinated outfit and others recognize and pay me a compliment no matter what my weight is."
-Cathy B., 66

"I feel most confident when I choose to be and when I treat myself well, both with my internal chatter and when I do things that make my body feel good (nutrition, movement, meditations)."
-Cherri J., 34

"When I am dressed in fancy clothes and shoes and have full makeup on and my hair is done."
-Heidi W., 44

Finally, what made a critical difference for many was what they were wearing (or not wearing) and the type of material and comfort of clothing they had on.

"When I am in my PJs, I feel incredible because my body is covered. I only feel comfortable when I feel thin."
-Jade B., 30

"When I've eaten in accordance with my body's needs. When I lift weights, do yoga and dance. When I wear clothes that are comfortable and accentuate my body in areas that I like. When I am NOT PMSing. When I've taken time to connect with my soul."
-Cydney P., 37

"Cotton makes me feel great as does exercise. And I absolutely love summer and summer clothes."
-Caren C., 56

"Jeans and a big, overhanging sweater or shirt."
-Anonymous

"I feel most comfortable in my skin in my favorite clothes—ones I feel I look good in while still being comfortable too."
-Bonnie M., 28

"In pajama flannel pants and a sweatshirt. Also, definitely when clothed, not naked. I feel comfortable walking outside or at the gym for exercise because it feels proactive and the clothing contains the shaking feeling of fat."
-Lisa P., 36

On the other hand, I wondered when people felt least comfortable in their skin and when were the times they literally wanted to crawl out of it. I cannot tell you how many people responded that they feel least comfortable when they need to wear a bathing suit and expose the parts of their bodies they are most insecure about in the public setting. I get that on a deep personal level and I think many women do. It wasn't until I was almost thirty years old that I even considered wearing a two-piece suit for the first time.

There is a poignant scene in a new TV series called "This is Us" that felled me emotionally on a deep and visceral level. I won't be spoiling the show by recounting this scene but will speak about it, because it truly encapsulates, for me, what so many young girls go through. What was most heartbreaking about the scene was that we, the audience, the millions of people watching, lay witness to this character understanding for the first time that her version of herself—the confident, beautiful and self-possessed person she naturally saw in herself—was different than those around her. The character, Kate, is a beautiful larger woman living in LA and navigating her chronic dieting world. She is trying to find herself, just like so many of us have. Through flashbacks, we are exposed to her journey from a happy, oblivious young girl to an insecure, body-loathing chronic dieter. This particular arc of the show profoundly moves me every time because of the nuanced vulnerability we see in her body image descent. Every time I see her character dealing with low self-esteem, I want to reach into the TV screen, hug her, and tell her how magnificently beautiful she is.

In this particular flashback, Kate is roughly ten years old and takes a trip to the local public pool with her family. She happily and innocently wears a bikini to the pool, despite being larger than many of the other kids, and refuses to bring a t-shirt, as her parents quietly plead with her to do so before leaving. Her parents are kind and care deeply about her, but they tacitly judge her, or at the very least, worry that she will be judged by others simply because of her size. Her "friends" at the pool snicker at her and ultimately send her a note saying they are embarrassed to play with her unless she covers up. Kate sulks sadly on her lounge chair and her parents find the note, leaving her loving dad to give her a pep talk and to lend her his t-shirt, but it's too late. The damage has been done. This was and will always be a seminal moment in her identity. She was body-shamed into covering up. We see through these flashbacks the very moment that defined Kate as a loather of her own body and so many of us can relate because we've had similar experiences.

An understanding about how shaming our bodies starts to unfold is witnessed before our very eyes through Kate's story. That this type of body-shaming remains today tells us how far we have to go in the movement of body positivity and health at every size. As long as unattainable body standards remain front and center in our purview via media, magazines, and even our role models, it will become increasingly hard to unshackle ourselves from dieting culture and mentality. I applaud "This is Us" for giving us a personal and unvarnished example of the very trajectory many girls face or faced growing up. There is no easy solution in the show or in real life to this monstrous problem, but that is okay as long as we are having the conversation.

QUESTION: *Can you describe when you feel LEAST comfortable in your skin or appearance (during Zumba, when presenting in front of other people, during sex, etc.)?*

"Pretty much all the time, except when I am alone."
-Anonymous

"In formal situations where the people who have "signature looks" really shine. You know those people who always look great, anywhere, because they have figured out the hairstyle and the clothing style and the pose that makes them look phenomenal, and who just work it all the time? I am NOT one of those people. I throw myself together every day, willy nilly. I had a professor in university single me out EVERY class to discuss my 'style' of the day. I am the furthest thing possible from having discovered my own 'look.' In nine out of ten situations, that doesn't matter at all in my life, but when I go to a fancy event where there are news cameras and such, I always feel unworthy of being there because... *What was I thinking wearing this dress or doing my hair like that or choosing this shade of lipstick, etc.?*"
-Monique M., 32

"Sex with a new partner."
-Anonymous

"Least comfortable when I'm on stage, in pictures, on video, anything where people are looking at me."
-Anita T., 51

"During exercise classes, in a swimsuit, out with friends who are thinner."
-Anonymous

"Honestly? When I'm around particularly negative or scrutinizing friends and family, and they turn their scrutinizing eyes on me."
-Sarah M., 24

"In a bathing suit at the beach. At least I go to the beach, because I have much thinner friends who will not even put on a bathing suit. I am not going to let my weight stop me from enjoying something I love so much."
-Cathy B., 66

"I would say, sometimes, when I tell people what I do or am trying to do in the health and wellness world, I feel that people sometimes expect someone in my role to be super skinny and super fit. It makes me feel uncomfortable and like I am being judged when all I want to do is help others."
-Erika S., 42

"When I am naked. When I have a pimple on my face. When I feel fat or overweight. I see crappy 'tagged' pictures of me on Facebook and I look terrible."
-Jade B., 30

Finally, I really wanted to hear from other people what it would take for them to love their bodies unconditionally. Was there some magic elixir one could take or would it require doing the hard work for a long time to bring respectfulness and kindness back with respect to their exteriors. Many people erroneously believe that once they are thin, they will be happy and fulfilled. They feel disillusioned and panicked when they realize that their thinness doesn't equate with happiness and that the work involved to stay thin makes being at their "ideal" body weight elusive for the long haul. Out of all the questions I asked the interviewees, this was the one where people struggled the most for answers. This is one of the reasons I knew this book was important to write and still relevant despite the work being done in the world of body positivity and the Health at Every Size movement.

QUESTION: *What do you believe it would take to love your body unconditionally?*

"That's an interesting question that I've never thought about in just this way before. I think it's mostly this really deep rooted, old belief that I won't be fully accepted or loved unless I look good. I've drastically shifted what my version of good is for myself and generally accept my body and don't tie my self-worth into it or feel that I need to look a certain way for others. But, it's definitely not completely gone, and when the question is posed, it comes up for me."
-Carly M., 39

"Interesting question. I'm not sure I ever would. I'd have to have the money to have laser eye surgery for my terrible vision, laser hair removal for legs and face, and laser rejuvenation treatment for my acne scars. (Looks like I should just buy my own laser!) But I can accept the imperfections. I just don't think you need to love the imperfections the same as you love the attributes."
-Marie P., 40

"I wish I knew. It is a work in progress. Part of the love is accepting that some days I will be less in love with my body than others."
-Anonymous

"I'm honestly not sure, besides realizing that how God sees me is most important and the rest doesn't matter, even if I have some "flaws." No one's body is perfect and that's part of what makes us unique."
-Bonnie M., 28

"Changing social standards so that our sense of self-worth isn't placed so heavily on something as transitory as physical appearance."
-Sarah M., 24

"A lot of therapy and to be deaf and blind to the negativity of others and the media's opinion of what beautiful is."
-Elizabeth S., 35

"This is a good question. I have been trying for my whole life, but it is hard to stop the negative self-talk sometimes. When I hear that negative self-talk creep in, I remind myself that I am strong, smart, and able to do whatever I set my mind to. The key is catching yourself in that moment."
-Erika S., 42

"I'm about as close to unconditional love for my body as I judge I can be. The only thing that I imagine would take me to 100%

complete, true unconditional love might be to hang out with Eckhart Tolle, The Dali Lama, and Ram Dass for a few years."
-Joe B., 35

"I don't know if I can ever do that... very sad."
-Lisa F., 66

"I don't think that I can. I don't know how any female can in this time."
-Heidi W., 44

"Getting into a healthy routine I enjoy. I am one for instant gratification. I feel like I have a habit of not committing and I constantly give up on things. I think I will be able to love myself if I reach a point where I find a hobby that I enjoy. Weird, right? Well, I've been without a hobby for two plus decades and haven't loved myself at all through them. I grew up taking care of others and I've spent the last few years trying to take care of me. Talk about DIFFICULT. I think once I reach a point of loving what I do, I will be able to focus less on shit that doesn't matter and more on what does matter. Me."
-Jade B., 30

"Continuing to do the healing work that I've spent the past two years doing. Every step is leading to a more powerful place in letting go of conditions and holding what is beautiful. I am no longer looking for THE perfect body. I'm looking to feel perfect in MY body!"
-Nikki B., 51

"Sadly, I don't know if I will ever really get there."
-Tami W., 40

"I think I'm pretty close now, despite what happened in my late teenage years. Maybe something to fix my breasts?"
-Talia K., 24

As you can see from these deeply personal and brave responses, the desire is there. There is a hunger to be unshackled from the many ways we convince ourselves that we aren't good enough as we are, but we just don't know how to do it.

When you read these quotes below, one cannot help but also feel stymied for answers and to empathize with the lack of insight that so many of us have in this area. This is the very reason we need a blueprint. A body image blueprint, if you will, to help get started in the hard work to follow. The work resides not only in each individual, but in society itself. When you have politicians who rate women between 1-10 on a scale of hotness, and celebrities who are criticized for the slightest imperfection, how can a little girl or a woman who is struggling every day to find deep acceptance crawl her way out of feeling the need to measure up? We, therefore, take on unsustainable and possibly unhealthy steps to attain this perfection.

In the next and last part of this book, we will explore the many techniques and tools that supported me in my journey toward body-acceptance and that I believe can help many others like myself.

PART III
THE BODY IMAGE
BLUEPRINT

"To love ourselves and support each other in the process of becoming real is perhaps the greatest single act of daring greatly."

—BRENÉ BROWN

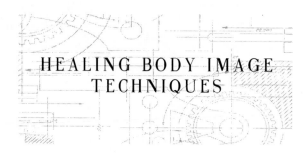

HEALING BODY IMAGE TECHNIQUES

I n the chapters that follow, we are going to explore many steps that you can start implementing right away. Some will give you immediate results, others will take a very long time to master, and still, others will take lifelong practice. Many of the body image healing strategies I talk about are well known and researched techniques, and were the very ideas I utilized to find my own healing and strength. Some of the tools are inspired by the tenets I learned at the Institute for the Psychology of Eating, while others are steps and techniques that I created and have implemented with my one-on-one clients. They are not meant to work in succession; you can pick and choose any that resonate with you. Some of you may need to utilize all of the steps in order to begin healing, and some may find what they need from just one or two. Try to see this as a time of exploration and self-discovery.

These strategies and ideas are not panaceas. The hard work and confrontation must be done slowly, persistently, and always with kindness and respect. Staying on the path is success. Staying engaged and always questioning the exterior, outdated societal beauty beliefs is success. Bringing yourself back to compassion and self-care, even when you hit setbacks, is success. Simply staying engaged is success. Try to be patient as you bring forth the courage to unfurl and unpeel the many layers of life experience that brought you here to this moment, reading this book. Be respectful of your story, your journey, and most importantly, of your own voice and inner wisdom. We will explore four body image realms:

The Embodiment Realm
The Physical Realm
The Social Realm
The Nutritional and Diet Realm

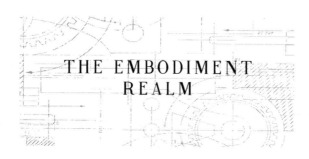

THE EMBODIMENT
REALM

The Embodiment Realm encompasses moving from the mind into the body. It includes embodiment work (which I'll discuss more below), gratitude practices, and mantras and mindfulness work around sensuality and sexuality. Many of us are uncomfortable being squarely in our bodies so we come up with clever ways to numb out or dissociate from our experiences in our bodies, especially if we hate the way we look or feel. The following techniques are designed to support the process from the cerebral to the physical. Because, as my mentor, Marc David, often said, it's when we "agree to be here," in our bodies, through thick and thin, through pain and pleasure, is when we can also begin the work of healing our body image.

EMBODY YOUR BODY

Have you ever been very deep in thought or involved in a quiet activity when suddenly, without notice, someone taps you on the shoulder? Your heart may race, you become solidly grounded in your body, and it's almost as if you went from head to body in a second flat. That is what it means to embody your body. Most of the time, we live in our heads and not our bodies. When bodily symptoms occur, such as a nagging cold or headache, we become aware of them but we take our meds and hope that we can soon be back in our thoughts. I'm not suggesting that we need to suffer or feel miserable. I do believe, however, that in order to fully appreciate the good, we need to experience and feel the bad. Many times, we hide or will away any uncomfortable symptoms in our bodies because it's easier to mask them than to really, really feel them.

When I experience anxiety, for example, I feel it all in my back—all the tension gets balled up there and stuck. For years, I took medicine and ignored it, trying to get back to my busy day. Now, I take a few minutes to do some deep breathing, some yoga and stretching, and sometimes even do a full workout. By getting into my body and out of my head, it dispels the anxiety more than anything I have ever done before.

Embodiment is a tool I use to also help people with body image challenges. Learning to be present in your body now, versus in the future when you will hopefully lose ten pounds, can only help you love and accept your body as it is right this very moment. Try out these embodiment techniques below.

Take a yoga class: These classes are designed to have you breathe, focus, and be completely aware in your body.

Thought bubble work: Try looking in the mirror and notice any negative self-talk thought bubbles that occur. Acknowledge and thank them, and continue to try to look without judgment. You can do this fully clothed, partially clothed, or naked. I suggest you attempt this for five to ten minutes at a time, a few times a week. The goal here is that by simply noticing the thought bubbles, acknowledging them and then letting them go, we can wade through the negative self-talk and notice the stories we tell ourselves about our bodies. Then, we can recognize that they are merely perceptions that we ascribe meaning to and not necessarily reality.

Go for a walk outside without distractions: Feel the wind on your face, notice the smells, and be aware of all of the sensations in and around you.

Do a five senses inventory: Pick out your favorite scented candle or perfume and take in the aroma. View nature. Eat your favorite food and savor every bite. Touch someone you love and have him or her touch you back. Listen to music and take in every note, every instrument, the tone of the singer's voice. Recognize what a blessing it is to be alive.

Do some deep stretching: Get to those tight, uncomfortable places and allow yourself to lean into and accept the discomfort fully before moving onto a new position.

Meditation: Notice your breath. It is the anchoring point in your body. From there, you can notice all other things going on within your body as well as your mind.

EMBRACE SENSUALITY AND SEXUALITY

I know this is a tough one for many. I also realize that sexuality and body image often go hand-in-hand. Some may read this and say, "I can't possibly feel good about sensuality and sexuality until I feel good in my body, lose weight, fit into a size ___, etc."

I respect that and fully understand, but I'm also kindly telling you to flip that notion on its head.

I'm suggesting that you should try standing out on the skinny branch and exploring these things, especially when you don't feel good about your body. Confront this head on, breathe through the discomfort and stay present, accepting, and forgiving of each thought or cringe that comes your way. I'm not a sexologist and I do not specialize in this area at all, but I do know that allowing yourself to feel the various sensations our bodies are capable of feeling can give you a sense of deep appreciation and respect for the amazing vessel your soul inhabits. Every body is capable of this.*

Start by simply exploring sensuality and take sex completely off the table. You can start alone, by just noticing what the feel of your hand is like on different parts of your body. You may notice that some places you touch, even gently, evoke strong emotions both good and bad. You can also experiment with different types of textures on the skin and different temperatures. You're becoming acquainted or reacquainted with your body and its responses to physical touch. Eventually, you can build up to exploring sensual touch with a partner who you know and completely trust. Gentle massage can be part of this exploration as well. Remember, there is no sexual component to this exercise; it's simply about noticing, observing, and eventually becoming more comfortable

*Please note that if you know or suspect that you experienced sexual trauma or abuse in your childhood or past, I do not recommend trying these methods. In these cases, it's best to work with a licensed psychotherapist and follow a specific treatment plan related to trauma.

with tactile experiences within your body. This part may take weeks or months until you are comfortable.

If and when you get to a point of feeling comfortable with sensuality, you can move into exploring sexuality, both alone and with a trusted partner. Practice mindful sex, if you will, by focusing on the breath and staying present in your body versus "checking out" or remaining stuck in unkind thought bubbles that may emerge that keep you from fully experiencing the moment.

BODY SCAN AND GRATEFULNESS SCAN

Because we spend so much time in our heads and not anchored in our bodies, we also end up "checking out" in other ways too, often eschewing the small whispers of communication our bodies give out to us all the time. Because we don't listen when the body whispers, we end up only paying attention when it is screaming, and then we look for the immediate intervention.

A daily body scan and gratefulness scan can get us in touch with our bodies and all the ways it talks to us on a regular basis. I prefer to do my scans first thing in the morning. It makes sense to try this when you are not hassled to be somewhere and you have a few minutes of relative quiet before the daily hustle begins. If mornings aren't the most peaceful time in your house, you can try doing this before bed instead. Similar to the sensuality practice, we're going to be using touch to get in tune with where your body is holding onto stress. I imagine my hands are full of warmth and kindness and that any part of my body that I touch will also be filled with kindness (I know this may be a bit woo-woo for some of you, but stick with me). I take deep breaths and notice what part of my body may be in discomfort or needs a little bit more compassion and kindness from me. For a long time, this was my stomach. I had always had a flat belly, and I originally felt angry and indignant that motherhood took that away from me. Now, I hold my tummy in great reverence for allowing me the gift of growing three children.

If you notice that you have pain or discomfort somewhere in particular, or that you feel resentful about a part of your body that is not perhaps cooperating with your desires of what it should look like or do, gently move your hands to that place and hold them there. Continue to take deep breaths and remain present, acknowledging whatever thoughts and feelings arise. After a few moments, determine the next place your warm, kind hands need to go. Repeat this exercise in all of the places that want a bit more love and attention. This does not need to be a long exercise; it can be done in ten minutes.

After going through the initial scan, take some time to visualize all the different parts of your body. Aim to find one thing you are grateful for about each part of your body. For instance, "I am grateful for my hands, which allow me to touch, write and grasp," or, "I am grateful for a strong back that holds me upright every day and carries my beautiful children for piggyback rides." You get the point. Stick with it, even if you are feeling negative and even if you are struggling with what to say.

We show gratitude for others daily, and now it's time to start showing gratitude for our own bodies that do so many amazing things for us every day.

REMEMBER WHAT YOUR SPECIFIC BODY PARTS ARE ACTUALLY FOR

When we are diet and appearance crazed, we may see our body parts as fat or freckled or full of veins or unattractive in some other way, completely forgetting that each part of our bodies was designed with purpose, to keep us safe and strong. When we can re-establish what our body parts are made to do, we can begin to respect and be in awe of ourselves. For instance, think about your arms for a moment. To the body-image challenged and appearance focused individual, those arms appear weak and flabby. To me, those arms represent what I use to hold my children, to carry the groceries, and to lift myself up into warrior pose in yoga. Do you see the distinction here? You can practice this with every part of your body that you have ever felt insecure about or uncomfortable with. Go ahead and give it a try.

POSITIVE MANTRAS AND AFFIRMATIONS

Piggybacking on the gratitude and body scan is giving yourself positive and self-affirming mantras to repeat throughout the day. They can be about your body but they can also be about food, movement, or even about facing challenges.

"I exercise to make me healthier, not skinnier."

....

"I make choices that nourish my body."

"I will not bully my body into something it doesn't want to be."

....

"I will respect my appetite today."

....

"I am much more than a number on a scale."

....

"I will be kind to my body today."

SPLURGE FOR A NUDE OR BOUDOIR PHOTO SHOOT

Trust me on this one. Do it for yourself and no one else. Yes, it will feel scary. Yes, you will be way out there on that skinniest of skinny branches in the depth of your discomfort. Yes, you will have imposter syndrome. Yes, you might feel awkward, but please believe me when I tell you that it will be worth every penny and every heart palpitation when you have those beautiful pictures in your hand and can see the depth of your sexiness, femininity, and beauty. If you are what I was like years ago, you think you look terrible in the present but then look back at old photos and wonder what on Earth you were so unhappy about. Why didn't you just appreciate where you were? We glorify the past and pine for the future, for a time when we will be happier, look different, lose those ten pounds, or fit into the skinny jeans again. What we don't realize is that our deepest happiness resides in this moment, right now. When we accept and love what is and take advantage of every moment, we take those feelings of gratitude with us into the future as we live and grow.

Do the boudoir shoot now! Don't wait until you've starved your way down another ten pounds or when you get that tummy tuck. Someday, you will look at the musty photos in your old age and smile to yourself with pride that you had the courage to face your fears, live in the present, and appreciate your beauty, no matter your size, weight, or age. When sampling this strategy, please do the research and interview several people to make sure you find someone who has a lot of experience and, most importantly, with whom you feel comfort and trust. Bring a friend or partner along as well for extra support if needed. Oh, and some wine never hurts either.

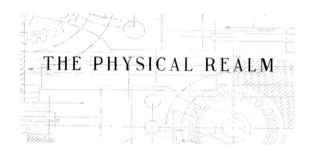

THE PHYSICAL REALM

The physical realm is similar to embodiment but with the specific goal of healing your potentially fraught relationship with exercise. If you have only known exercise and physical movement as a means to an end for weight loss then exploring these strategies may be very eye opening and healing for you.

GET YOUR OM ON!

I always felt yoga was something I should do, even though I felt uninspired and bored the times I had tried it. Remember, cardio was king to me at the time I had first experimented with yoga, therefore, I saw no point in doing it. Later on, when I tried hot yoga, a profound turnaround occurred for me and I was hooked. Not only was it cardio-based but yoga also challenged me with flexibility, balance, and mental focus. I know hot yoga or Bikram yoga is not for everyone, but I love it for several reasons:

1) When it is very hot in the room, I am forced to stay present to all the experiences, good and bad, that are happening in the moment.

2) I cannot daydream during hot yoga and must be mindful. This keeps me in tune with my breath, which is at the very core of calming myself down during a difficult pose, calming my heart rate, and giving me confidence that I can get through that blasted five-count from the instructor.

3) I see tangible growth and change each week, albeit subtle, which gives me confidence in myself and an appreciation for the strength and resiliency that resides within me. It's pretty powerful stuff.

I recall one very difficult hot yoga class I was in, where it literally felt like it was 150 degrees in there. Each time I thought we were getting a child's pose break, she'd have us doing some acrobatic feat instead. Halfway through the class, I felt completely spent and I wanted to leave. It was almost as if she had been reading my energy because the next sentence out the instructor's mouth was this: "You may be feeling deep discomfort right now, but I want you to know that you have everything you need within your well of strength to get through this moment and get through this class. You have all the self-soothing and calming techniques available to you to tap into right now and it starts with your breath." She was right. I did have it within me, but I felt unwilling to tap into it and come up against "my edge" as she described it.

Once I tapped into this strength, I was able to finish out the class with a sense of bliss and accomplishment. I thanked my body for what it had achieved and felt the level of trust within my body increase considerably that day. This is what yoga can do for men and women who struggle with body image. It is an extremely useful practice and everyone should give it a chance.

Action Item:

Research yoga studios in your area. Start with a basic class and work your way up. There are so many different types of yoga: vinyasa flow, Bikram, gentle yoga, hatha yoga, and lots of hybrids. Sample many of them and see which type suits you best. Alternatively, you can sign up for Gaiam TV, which live streams yoga classes and allows you to start from the comfort of your home. There are also yoga instructors that come to your home for private lessons if that intrigues you.

OTHER ENERGY WORK TO EXPLORE:
Reiki
Mindfulness Meditation
EFT
CBT Therapy
Body Positive Retreats
Acupuncture
Massage
Qigong

INCORPORATE JOY AND PLAY INTO YOUR EXERCISE ROUTINE

I have talked at length in this book about my conflicted relationship with exercise and how I transitioned from exercising because I felt I had to in order to punish myself for the cake I ate the previous night, to exercising my body because I absolutely enjoyed doing it. This took time. It took a commitment to a new path and, ultimately, a paradigm shift within my understanding of the purpose of movement. I determined that exercise is biologically intrinsic to our health and that the very nature of the techno-logical society we currently live in pretty much voids our will to move every day. The advent of elevators, escalators, online shopping, and even remote controls all serve to take us further away from spontaneous and natural movement. The more sedentary we became, the more we had to rely on creative measures to move our bodies. We went from walking to school and work to joining fancy gyms and hiring personal trainers.

My path led me from over-exercising on machines to exploring natural movement progressions in my body related to my own bodily mechanics and the ways that I find pleasure in movement. This was the game-changer for me. It was a pure revelation to know I could burn just as many calories play-wrestling with my husband as I could from chugging away mindlessly and painfully on an elliptical. I could hike and explore nature. I could go dancing. I could play Red Light, Green Light 123 with my kids and that all counts! I could do five ten-minute bouts of walking as opposed to pushing myself on a busy day to find one solid hour, and that counts too.

Most importantly, I got back in touch with the ways I like to move my body. That movement might be completely different than someone else's version, and I get to discover daily where my inner athlete resides and where I find my strength. My challenge to you is to do the same. I used to scoff at any exercise class or plan that wasn't keen on heavy cardio. Now I know that it all counts and it all matters.

Action Item:

Think of the games, sports, or ways you enjoyed moving as a child. Was it a rousing game of Monkey in the Middle? Was it riding your bike? Was it running and jumping into a pool? Was it climbing the monkey bars at the playground? Write down a list of all the ways you moved as a kid and what you particularly enjoyed about it. Next, tackle one of those items per week, even if you feel really silly doing it. When you get back in touch with play and joy as it relates to movement, it enables you to embody your body during exercise again rather than numbing out by watching the Food Network on the elliptical. It also allows you to appreciate and respect the non-linear ways we can move rather than the cookie cutter approaches that so many exercise programs espouse.

You can make up any others that specifically resonate for you, based on your own situation.

*Before starting any exercise regime, please consult a physician. Also, hot yoga may not be right for everyone, especially if you have or have had anorexia and other eating disorders.

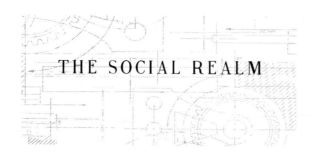

THE SOCIAL REALM

A s I've discussed several times in this book, our perception of what a "normal" body looks like is often informed by external sources such as our parents, our peers, strangers, and even our teachers or other authority figures. Those are important influences, but it's important to note that what we see on TV, in magazines and movies, or on social media can be the most persuasive of all. This is because it is so persistently in our faces.

TAKE A MEDIA/MAGAZINE/REALITY TV HIATUS

How can a young child not slowly perceive themselves as different and potentially not as worthy when they realize that they don't look like the perfect men and women in the magazines? As a tween, I would watch soap operas and make the connection that if I looked like the women in the show then I, too, would attract the hot guy and have everything I want in life. Whether the mode of communication was subtle or extremely blatant, the message was always clear: Thinness and beauty meant power. The same was true about my teen bop magazines and movies I watched. My "role models" in the eighties were Christie Brinkley, Cindy

Crawford, and Julia Roberts. Did the ordinary woman of average height with varicose veins, droopy breasts, and a post-baby bump ever get featured getting the hot guy at the end? Not that I recall.

Media saturation can have a poignant and lasting effect on our psyches and infuse us with messages that we must change our bodies and our natural appearance if we are ever to be worthy of love and acceptance. Try this experiment: Find two or three magazines you read and circle every example of a woman or man who looks kind of perfect. Notice what they are selling. Make a list of ten examples of this. By the end, you should see ten products or services that you absolutely must buy if you would like to look as good as the photoshopped woman or man in the ad. Everywhere you look, someone is reminding you that you are not good enough the way you are.

How do we combat this? I recommend taking a hiatus from the fashion magazines, reality TV, and any social media that you notice promoting "perfect" bodies and doesn't include every day women and men that you would see on the street. Even if it's for a day, notice where these messages are coming from and take a time out from them. Reflect on how you feel after a brief hiatus, and then possibly move to the next step.

JOIN SOCIAL NETWORKS THAT EMBRACE BODY-POSITIVITY AND HEALTH AT EVERY SIZE

When I was deep in my confusion about whether to conform to dieting culture in order to achieve the pyrrhic victory of thinness or to buck the trend with a huge middle finger, I had no idea resources existed that spoke exactly to me and who I was! Since I decided to officially end my career in dieting, my eyes have been opened to the vast networks out there that support people to rise above body-shaming by promoting a place of body acceptance and positivity. These resources have helped me immensely and they can do the same for you too. These networks inspired me to host a screening of the movie Embrace, which features an array of self-affirming, body-positive, and diverse stories from women and men around the world with activist Taryn Brumfitt at the helm, ushering us through and reminding us along the way of her own powerful and brave story. Hosting the movie for 100 people in Boston on a Monday night was a powerful culmination of my life's work up to that point, and it was heartening to see the positive response. Here are some body-positive resources for you to begin exploring:

Body Image Movement
About Face
A Beautiful Body Project
The Body Positive
Beauty Redefined
About that Curvy Life
Be Nourished
A Year Without Mirrors
Sarah Berneche

Some great Facebook groups to join to get more positivity in your Facebook feeds:

Curvy Confidence with Natalie Baack
Taryn Brumfitt fan page
Body Love Wellness
Break the Rules: Body Positive and Anti-Diet Community with Summer Innanen

And here are some wonderful podcasts for you to consider that can further enhance and entrench you into body-positivity and away from body-shaming:

The Love, Food Podcast
Food Psych Podcast
The F*ck It Diet Radio
Body Bliss
Psychology of Eating Podcast
The Everyday Woman Podcast (I'm featured on this one – episode #5)
Fearless Rebelle Radio
Let It Out with Katie Dalebout

ASSOCIATE YOURSELF WITH SUPPORTIVE, NON-JUDGMENTAL PEOPLE

Disassociate with diet-obsessed, appearance-focused, and otherwise judgmental people.

Please don't misunderstand me. I don't want you to go out and ditch all of your long-standing friends. What I am suggesting is that it is only to your benefit if you choose to be around people who do not keep you in dieting mentality. I had a friend who I really liked hanging out with and we were friends for several years. What I realized over time, however, is that I always felt insecure about my looks around her. I felt that I had to dress in a certain way to impress her and I always left our encounters feeling quite drained. When I pondered this further, I realized that this woman was always commenting on other people's appearances—so and so had gained some weight, so and so looks amazing in her yoga pants. There was an air of scrutiny in everything she talked about. I knew that it was only a matter of time before she was talking about me in some way or another. Even though she was nice and fun to be around, I made the choice to disassociate with her because I didn't need to feel the additional pressure of inadequacy. I generated plenty of that myself.

This woman and I are still acquaintances and I don't go out of my way to avoid her, but I'm much happier being around my more laid back, soul-focused friends instead. The ones that lift me up and love me unconditionally are the people who fuel my tank and don't leave me feeling depleted at the end of a hang out.

If you don't have people in your life like this, seek them out. Befriend them. Find your unabashed, body-celebrating tribe. Until you find them, feel free to use me as your surrogate! Join my "Wellness Warriors" Facebook group and find 1000+ like-minded people who are also slowly getting released from dieting culture.

THE NUTRITION AND DIETARY REALM

I t's very cliché to tell people to "eat clean," or to instruct people to obey an organic, whole foods based diet. Most people know this is best and everyone wants to eat this way, but they still don't really know how to make it work. The most common request I get from my clients is for me to just tell them what to eat. I understand it, and I wish it were as easy as an exchange of words between a client and myself. Instead, what I work on with clients is getting back in touch with sensuality around their food choices, slowing down and making food decisions based on their own intrinsic wisdom. You don't see lions in the wild, ruminating whether they should eat the antelope or the zebra that day, or if they should cut back on the wild hogs so they can be svelte enough for the lion cotillion later that month. Yet, human beings struggle with their food choices and with using their internal wisdom every day.

FINDING YOUR 50 SHADES OF GREY WITH FOOD

Finding your way to healthy food and balance after years of a binge/restrict mentality is not easy. I get that. When clients tell me that they never crave vegetables, I answer with a resounding,

"Of course you don't! You have years of eating processed foods or forcing yourself to eat foods you think you should only because it's healthy. Why on Earth would you crave foods you don't think you like?" It's a vicious cycle. The very act of restricting or denying ourselves food makes us yearn for those foods with a vengeance.

The first technique I utilize with my clients is to have them put all food on the table. Nothing is off limits. This makes them visibly uncomfortable at first because they are so used to rules and regulations and structure. They fear that being let off the leash will result in massive weight gain and constant consumption of junk food. Once they get past this, a wonderful pathway opens to them to decide for themselves what to eat and how much of it to eat.

After so many years of denying, there will, indeed, be some overeating of the "forbidden" foods, but they know they have me as a safety net and anchor. Once that initial binge is laid to rest, people find they truly want to eat healthy foods and start to seek it out. Concurrently, I work to implement mindful eating practices with my clients and walk them through how to eat a piece of chocolate, for instance, using all of their senses. I also provide resources and recipes to help them start incorporating healthy foods into their diet, always on their own terms. With continued mindful eating, clients discover for themselves that the very foods they were addicted to, now make them feel sick and don't taste nearly as good as they once did. Think of the personal power there. There is no outside expert telling them what to eat. It's all coming from within.

When people make internal, intuitive decisions about how to nourish their body, they are also sending a wink and a nod to their body that it's okay to trust itself again. They start to trust that there will no longer be any self-induced famine or disrespect. The body responds in kind, making them feel better, giving them more energy, and maybe even starting to losing weight slowly and naturally. The idea is to love and respect the body into the weight you're supposed to be rather than bullying it there. From that place, a healthy relationship is able to blossom between you and your body.

MORE ON MINDFUL EATING

People who have challenges with body image often also have a fraught relationship with food as well, or at the very least, a polarizing and conflicting relationship with food. When you can focus on being aware, present and mindful during the eating experience, many doors of reflection can open up for you. First and foremost, you begin to get out of the head and into the body during the eating experience to understand better what food fuels you, how much of it makes you feel good and energized, and at what point you feel fatigue or overfull. It's hard to figure all of that out when you're eating in your car or watching TV, furtively chowing ding-dongs while standing up and pretending it's not happening.

Mindful eating is about respect; respect for understanding your appetite, your proclivities around food, and yes, around your body. Knowing when to stop eating because you are satisfied sets the tone for being respectful in other ways around your body as well. All good relationships are based on trust, respect, and communication. Learning the basic tenets of mindful eating affords you all three of those important facets necessary for a successful relationship with yourself. To get started, try these four strategies:

Action Item:

1) Aim to take five to ten deep, grounding breaths before eating anything.

2) Put your food on a plate and sit down at the table, without distraction, fully owning your decision to eat your chosen food at that moment.

3) Chew your food five to ten times between bites to allow for full mastication of your food and important enzymatic processes to occur, courtesy of your salivary glands.

4) Put your fork or spoon down between bites.

Action Item:

Try putting all your diet books and online diet challenges away for a month and unsubscribe from all the diet experts that show up in your inbox. Put the scale in a locked drawer and fully feel the discomfort of not having that particular tool to tell you how you did that week. You know what your week was like, much more than the scale does! Without this external crutch, you will be forced to trust the decisions you made and the behaviors you did on any day instead of a hunk of metal giving you a subjective pass or fail. I'm not saying you should never weigh yourself again. Just give it a month where you completely trust and obey the signals your body sends as to how it wants to be fed and nourished. Honor your appetite and cues. Try using tools rather than rules with respect to eating healthy. Create healthy systems, like carrying bags of raw veggies with you or keeping trail mix in your handbag for when you're hungry on-the-go, rather than forcing yourself to eat at a certain time or forcing yourself NOT to eat at other times simply because of a rule you learned in a diet book.

DISCOVER FOODS THAT MAKE YOU FEEL WONDERFUL IN YOUR SKIN

The perfect diet for my body may be completely different than yours. Luckily, we have the kind of variety in food that allows for us both to thrive, feel amazing in our skin, and nourish ourselves adequately. I often counsel clients to choose foods that are balanced based on the macronutrient trifecta of lean proteins, healthy fats, and complex carbohydrates. This gives them a compass without me actually telling them what to eat. There are infinite ways to create healthy meals with this credo in mind. In the appendix section, you will see several recipes that comport to this philosophy.

Part of healing our body image requires finding the very foods that make our bodies feel good and to respect our bodies by feeding them exactly what they are asking for. Eating healthy fats is often the most difficult for body image challenged clients. For far too long we have been fed the myth that the fat in our food is the cause of weight gain and high cholesterol. My clients happily chow down on full-fat yogurt, avocado, nuts and seeds, and salmon, and find that they feel healthier, more satiated and happier than ever.

Action Item:

Here are some examples of mixed and matched foods that give you macronutrient balance and the opportunity to have your body feel its best. Please sample a few combinations and a recipe or two from the the end of this book.

Healthy Fats Examples:
- High quality oils, like olive, sesame, coconut, macadamia nut, sunflower, flax, almond, walnut
- High quality nuts and seeds, raw and organic
- Olives
- Wild fish, especially salmon
- Free-range eggs
- High quality butter
- High quality dairy that is organic, hormone-free, especially full-fat Greek yogurt
- Coconut

Complex Carbohydrates:
- Fruits
- Vegetables
- Brown rice
- Whole grain bread
- Whole grain pasta
- Quinoa
- Teff, sorghum, and other ancient grains
- Whole grain cereals, including steel cut oats
- Legumes, like chickpeas, lentils, navy beans, black-eyed peas

Lean Protein Examples:
- white fish
- salmon, tuna, or other dark fish
- skinless chicken or turkey
- lean ground beef or turkey

- veggie burger
- tofu
- egg whites or eggs
- tempeh
- beans
- pork
- lamb
- shellfish
- Greek yogurt
- cottage cheese
- other soft and hard cheeses
- nut butter
- nuts or seeds

Examples of Mix & Match Meals & Snacks:
- Haddock with broccoli and brown rice
- Ezekiel bread with smashed avocado and turkey slices
- Whole wheat pasta with chicken, asparagus, and olive oil
- Apple with unsweetened almond butter or peanut butter
- Quinoa with seeds and vegetables

MICRO-STRATEGIES

- Accept compliments fully and without a response other than, "Thank you." Look the person in the eye and say "thank you" in a sincere way. Accepting compliments and letting them wash over you is a form of self-love and acceptance.

- Challenge yourself to do things that are uncomfortable to you. Take on challenges that get you out of your comfort zone, but not into your stress/unattainable zone. Feeling a sense of accomplishment through hard work and effort gives you an appreciation for what you are capable of when you step out on the skinny branch. But it also serves as a conduit to self-appreciation and self-love. In fact, there is nothing more grounding and humbling than working hard, failing, trying again and again, and then accomplishing something. It allows for compassion and understanding that others may struggle in some ways too.

- Explore expressing all pillars of who you are—examine your hobbies, passions, community, social circles, relationships, spirituality, and make sure you are as balanced and in alignment as possible.

- Write a happiness inventory and add at least one item per day.

- Be in nature. There is nothing more humbling than being in the wilderness and recognizing that we are just specks in this vast, amazing world. It also helps to put our corporeal concerns in perspective. Additionally, being in nature is a wonderful method for practicing mindfulness.

- Explore bodies of water. Our bodies feel different in water than on land. Enjoy the sense of lightness and expansiveness in various pools, oceans, lakes, and hot tubs.

- Journal and write about the experience of being in your body. Write daily, even if only a few sentences.

- Write a letter to your body. What would you say to it? What might it write back to you in response?

OUR GIRLS AND BOYS ARE LISTENING—WHAT WILL WE SAY?

We live in a diet-obsessed culture where we regularly witness the descent of beautiful, strong girls into yo-yo dieting, hatred of their bodies, and sometimes into lifelong struggles with eating disorders and body dysmorphia. While I am one of the lucky ones who was finally able to pull the curtain in time to heal and change and grow into the person I was meant to be, there is no guarantee that others will follow. I feel a sense of deep obligation to keep this conversation going and to unpeel the stubborn and stinging layers of our personal onions, to understand whose voice is guiding these beliefs and, ultimately, behaviors that end up causing us so much angst.

As the mom of three young girls, I feel both trepidation and relief that I am at the helm of their own body image journeys. For one, there is only so much a mom can do. I have hopefully laid sturdy foundations of self-acceptance and pride about who they are as people, irrespective of how they look, but I know my influence is fleeting. Soon, powerful outside forces will whisk them away on a separate journey; one that they will have to navigate mostly on their own through thorns and thistles. They will need to find their own voices outside the clutter of media, peers, and potential romantic partners.

What we must continue to do as a society is question the notion that only certain bodies are beautiful and others are not. The idea that we must spend money, time, our precious energy and resources to change who we are in order to be loved and accepted must be dismantled. We have to do the hard work of confronting these injustices as they occur and buck against them every step of the way. There are no easy answers or solutions. We all must put in the hard work.

When you think about the end of your life, do you want to say you spent your days obsessing and worrying about your weight and appearance, or that you lived your life on your own terms, spent time with those you loved, and pursued your passions and dreams with gumption? I think you know the answer to this. Now it's up to you to follow through. Use this book as your jumping off point for your own body image blueprint; one that can be left as a compass for your own children and generations to come.

Listening to your body is important, but if these strategies feel impossible or overwhelming to you, that is okay. It may mean that you might need to seek professional support. I recommend MEDA if you live in the Boston area and NEDA nationally to find an eating disorder specialist.

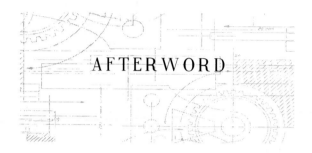

AFTERWORD

About a year after launching my business, honing and getting my message about body positivity, anti-dieting and eating psychology out to the world, I received some surprising hate mail. This email took my breath away in its ignorance and cruelty, and I needed to take some time to process it and how I would react. Here's the content of the email:

> "How can someone as hugely fat as you be talking about teaching weight loss and a healthy relationship to food???? What kind of deep denial are you in? Have you seen your own pictures?"

Even seeing these words again now, as I write them, makes my heart skip a beat. When I first received the anonymous note, it was very triggering for me. I was instantly catapulted back to the narrative I had described throughout this book. Part of me wanted to diet like a fiend, just for this one internet troll, to prove to her I was not an imposter. Another part of me wanted to write back and tell her to fuck off! And still, another part of me wanted me to point out her ignorance, explain what my mission is really about, and have her understand how hurtful her words were. I did none of the above. I ignored her.

Here's the thing, though. My husband, my best friends, and some mentors that I shared this email with at the time told me that receiving this is actually a good thing. It's good because I hit a nerve in this person.

When I was initially destroyed and emotionally reeling from this email, my dear friend, Abby (the figurative nudes photographer), wrote this email to console me.

I really can't say it better than this:

If someone took the time and energy to write something so base, so vulgar, so spiteful - this person has a lot of self-hatred. No self-respecting individual would aim to cut down another person so sharply. Behind the veil of anonymity, this troll - let's call it what it is, Jenny - is looking to lash out his or her anger on an individual that appears to have it together. Never mind the fact that you doubt yourself at times. That's normal and expected. Think about your presence online: you have EMBRACED! You are vehemently body-positive, self-accepting, and possess an incredibly healthy relationship with food and with your gorgeous curves. You exude confidence and promote self-love - everything this person probably lacks in his or her own life. There will always, ALWAYS be trolls, girl. When there are naysayers, that means that you're effective. You're touching a nerve, inciting a reaction. This person, who has so much self-loathing and vitriol, is upset that you have achieved something s/he has not: peace with one's self. In art, we always rejoice at any reaction, whether positive or negative. A reaction means that someone has heard you. Take this person's venom not as any indication of your own body image or self-worth, but as a sign that your journey has affected others.

Some people who lack self-love feel the need to harm anyone who possesses that vital attitude. That is a reflection on them, not on you. This person is a bully. This person is spewing empty language, and is using it as a fig leaf for his/her own doubt, fear, anger, and dysmorphia.

When you look at your picture, what do you see? I see someone who is full of vitality, spunk, and fervor. I see courage, exoticism (oh yes!), and strength. I see a powerful woman who is at the top of her game and is reaching out her arms to bring others up with her. You already have gone high, girl.

There is no need for a response to this troll. If you do need to say something, which you might, turn it into a teachable moment. This kind of language is hurtful - to others, and especially to ourselves. How many women say the same horrible things to themselves when they look in the mirror each day? It's time to divorce ourselves of this judgment. It's time to embrace our bodies, which are healthy, energetic, able, and strong.

You know what? Let's bring this back to the OG (original goddess {sic}), Taryn Brumfitt. She received countless hate messages when she first started her positivity campaign. What did Taryn do? She didn't prove herself to anyone. She didn't offer an explanation. There was no need. She kept on doing what she was doing. You, too, will keep going. You will use your wit, creativity and passion to stand against hostility and shaming. You will embrace, and you will triumph.

I love you so much, Jenny. You are fucking incredible, and you are making a difference.

This book. This is my teachable moment. Let's all make a difference. Let's keep the conversation going.

....

RECIPES TO MAKE YOUR BODY FEEL HEALTHY AND BALANCED

The recipes listed here are all vegetarian recipes simply because that is what works for me and aligns with my beliefs and lifestyle. If you would like more specific guidelines on how to incorporate animal-based or other types of recipes, please consult with a registered dietician for support.

AVOCADO TOAST WITH SALSA

Avocados are my favorite snack ever. I used to shy away from them because I was worried about their fat content, but now I know better. Now I know that it's this very kind of fat that our bodies need to feel full and satisfied and that so many of us lack in our diets! While my favorite avocado recipe is guacamole, avocado toast is a close second. This recipe is amazing and is a delicious, balanced meal or snack that you can make very easily and in little time. Enjoy!

Serves 1
Recipe by: Arlene Jacobs

Ingredients:
1 slice whole grain bread, toasted
¼ ripe avocado, slightly mashed
2 tbsp salsa, hot or mild
1 hardboiled egg, chopped
Parsley or cilantro sprigs (optional)
Salt, to taste

Method:
Top toasted bread with mashed avocado, salsa, and sprinkle with chopped egg. Season to taste and serve with parsley or cilantro.

MUESLI WITH STRAWBERRIES, BLUEBERRIES AND YOGURT

Serves 2
Recipe by: Arlene Jacobs

Ingredients:
1 cup old-fashioned rolled oats
½ cup orange juice
¼ cup almond milk or skim milk
¼ cup yogurt (or substitute 1/8 cup almond milk for vegan)
½ unpeeled shredded apple
1½-2 tbsp honey
2 tbsp dark raisins
¼ cup almonds, roughly chopped
½ tsp lemon juice, or to taste
Strawberries
Blueberries
Yogurt

Method:
Combine all ingredients in a bowl and refrigerate overnight. Serve with berries and yogurt.

NOTE: You can substitute any nuts for muesli and/or cut-up fruits for topping.

SPINACH/FETA POLENTA PIE

Everyone loves pie of some kind, right? For me, beyond the apple, cherry and pecan favorites, there is something about a salty, savory pie that is very comforting and delicious. The creaminess of polenta coupled with the salty bite of feta marries very well in this dish. You're even upping your iron levels here with a good helping of spinach to boot.

Serves 4
Recipe by: Arlene Jacobs

Ingredients:

2 tbsp plus 1 tsp extra virgin olive oil
5 oz baby spinach
4 scallions, white and green parts, chopped
2 tbsp chopped dill
2 tbsp chopped parsley
Salt & pepper, to taste
3 cups vegetable broth
1 cup instant polenta
¼ cup grated parmesan cheese
3/4 cup crumbled feta cheese, plus extra for garnish

Method:

Over medium-high, heat 2 tbsp of the oil in a 10-11 inch skillet. Add the spinach, scallions, dill and parsley. Season with salt and pepper and sauté, tossing frequently for about 5 minutes.

In a medium saucepan, bring 3 cups vegetable broth to a boil and add the polenta in a steady stream, stirring constantly. When the polenta begins to thicken, add the parmesan and ½ cup of the feta cheese and stir until melted. Add salt and pepper, as necessary.

Pour the thickened polenta into an ovenproof serving dish, which has been greased with 1 tsp olive oil, and spread evenly. Top with the spinach mixture and sprinkle with remaining feta cheese. Drizzle with the remaining olive oil. Heat for about 20 minutes. Sprinkle with fresh herbs and serve.

NOTE: Serve with fresh figs and kalamata olives.

PORTOBELLA SLOPPY JOES

As a vegetarian for many years, I appreciate that there is something very "meaty" and *umami*-ish (is that a word?) about portobella mushrooms, in particular, that is very satisfying to me. Try serving them with baked potato wedges.

Serves 4.
Recipe by: Arlene Jacobs

Ingredients:
4 medium portobella caps
Salt & pepper, to taste
3 tbsp olive oil
4 rosemary sprigs
2 cups onions, diced
1 cup red peppers, diced
3 cups kidney beans, drained
3/4 cup quinoa, cooked
3 tbsp ketchup
2 tsp Dijon mustard
1 tsp Worcestershire sauce
½ tsp garlic powder

Method:
Preheat oven to 400°F.

Sprinkle the portobella caps with salt and pepper, to taste, and rub all over with 1 tbsp of the olive oil. Place each on a small sheet pan or ovenproof skillet. Slip a rosemary sprig under each cap.

Cover loosely with foil and bake for 20 minutes. Turn off heat and let mushrooms rest in the warm oven.

In a large skillet, sauté the onions and red peppers in the remaining 2 tbsp of olive oil until soft, about 5 minutes. Add the kidney beans, mix and mash slightly with the onions and peppers. Add the quinoa, ketchup, mustard, Worcestershire sauce, and garlic powder. Season with salt and pepper, to taste. Continue to cook, stirring occasionally for about 10 minutes. Add some water if mixture becomes too dry.

Mound the Sloppy Joe mixture on a plate and top with the mushroom caps.

CUCUMBER/MINT SELTZER (AKA MOCK MOJITO)

Serves 1
Recipe by: Arlene Jacobs

Ingredients:
2-inch piece of cucumber, seeded and finely chopped
4 mint leaves
1 tsp lime juice
½ tsp simple syrup
6 oz seltzer (approximately)

Simple Syrup Method:
In a small saucepan, combine a ½ cup of sugar and a ½ cup of water, stir, bring to a boil. Lower heat and simmer until all the sugar has dissolved. Let cool and store in the refrigerator for several weeks. Use as needed.

Place the chopped cucumber and mint into a tall 8 oz glass. Use the handle of a wooden spoon muddle to break up and bruise the mint and cucumber. Add 4-5 ice cubes, the lime juice, and simple syrup. Stir.

TOFU "STEAKS" WITH SMOKED PAPRIKA AIOLI

Serves 4
Recipe by: Arlene Jacobs

Ingredients:
Brine:
2 cups water
½ cup kosher salt
1 tbsp sugar

Tofu:
1 lb extra firm tofu, cut into 5/8-inch planks
1 tsp dried oregano
2 tsp garlic powder
2 tbsp Worcestershire sauce
½ tsp ground black pepper
1/2 cup corn starch
2 tbsp extra virgin olive oil
¼ cup parsley, chopped

Method:
In a small pot, combine the water, salt, and sugar and heat on medium-high until salt and sugar are dissolved. Let cool, place tofu planks in a shallow container and pour over the brine to cover. Allow tofu to macerate for 15 minutes.

Remove tofu and place between paper towels to dry. Sprinkle on both sides with the oregano, garlic powder, black pepper, and Worcestershire. Rub to blend.

Heat extra virgin olive oil over medium-high heat. Spread the cornstarch on a shallow plate, dredge the tofu thoroughly in the cornstarch, and pat between hands to remove excess cornstarch. Place in the pan and sauté for about five minutes on each side until golden brown.

Serve immediately over greens of choice and sprinkle with parsley. Serve smoked paprika aioli on the side.

Smoked Paprika Aioli:
½ cup mayonnaise
¼ cup yogurt
3/4 tsp lemon juice
½ tsp smoked paprika
Salt, to taste
3-5 drops Tabasco sauce
Stir together to combine

QUINOA WITH TRI-COLORED ROASTED CARROTS, SWISS CHARD, AND PISTACHIOS

Serves 4-6
Recipe by: Jenny Berk

Ingredients:

1 cup quinoa
3 each of purple, orange, and yellow carrots, ¼" bias cut
2 cups vegetable broth or water
¼ cup plus 2 tbsp olive oil
2 cups Swiss chard
Juice of one lemon
1 tbsp lemon zest, grated
1 tsp garlic powder
1 tbsp Dijon mustard
2 shallots, chopped
½ cup pomegranate seeds
½ cup of pistachios, chopped
Parsley, chopped
Salt & pepper, to taste

Method:

Preheat oven to 400°F.

Cook the quinoa as indicated on the box, using vegetable broth or water. Set aside in a large serving bowl.

Arrange carrots on a baking sheet. Add 2 tbsp of the oil, season with salt, pepper, and a teaspoon of garlic powder and mix to combine. Bake the vegetables for 40-45 minutes, turning and tossing once at the halfway point.

Rinse the Swiss chard, roll, and slice it into ribbons.

In a medium bowl, add the mustard, lemon juice, zest, shallots, salt and pepper. Slowly drizzle in the olive oil while stirring with a whisk to create an emulsion.

Add the roasted vegetables and Swiss chard to the quinoa and toss with the dressing. Check seasonings. Before serving, garnish the dish with the pistachios, pomegranate seeds, and chopped parsley.

YELLOW BEET AND BLOOD ORANGE SALAD

Serves 4
Recipe By: Arlene Jacobs

Ingredients:
2 large yellow beets
2 blood oranges
1 tsp orange zest
½ bunch asparagus
4 tbsp extra virgin olive oil
½ tsp Dijon mustard
2 tsp lemon juice
1 tbsp orange marmalade
1 tbsp shallots, chopped
Salt & pepper, to taste
¼ cup pistachios, chopped
1 cup mixed sprouts

Method:
Preheat the oven to 400°F.

Wash the beets, cut off both the root and stem ends, and wrap them in foil. Roast for about 1 hour, until soft in the middle when pierced with a knife. Let cool. Peel and cut into 3/8" rounds.

Wash and trim the tough ends of the asparagus, place on a sheet pan, and drizzle with 1 tbsp of the extra virgin olive oil. Season with salt and pepper. Roast uncovered for 5-7 minutes. Let cool.

Wash and peel the blood oranges and cut them into 3/8" rounds.

In a small bowl, add the Dijon mustard, lemon juice, marmalade, salt and pepper. Whisking constantly, slowly add the remaining 3 tbsp olive oil until well combined. Stir in orange zest.

Arrange the beets, oranges, and asparagus on the plate and sprinkle them with the pistachios. Sprinkle lightly with salt and pepper. Garnish the plate with the sprouts and drizzle everything with the vinaigrette.

PICADILLO TOFU STUFFED PEPPERS

Serves 4
Recipe by: Arlene Jacobs

Ingredients:
2 tbsp extra virgin olive oil
3 large green peppers, 2 cut in half, seeds removed, one chopped
1 large Spanish onion, chopped
4 cloves garlic, finely chopped
1 lb extra firm tofu, drained and crumbled
1½ tsp cumin
1½ tsp cinnamon
1 Turkish bay leaf
1-2 pinches cayenne
1 pinch ground cloves
1½ cups tomatoes, chopped (from carton or can)
1 tbsp cider vinegar
½ cup dark raisins
½ cup green pitted olives, rinsed and roughly chopped
Salt & pepper, to taste

Method:
Preheat oven at 400°F.

Heat the olive oil in an 11" or 12" sauté pan over medium-high, sauté the chopped green peppers and onions for 6-8 minutes, stirring occasionally until translucent.

Add the garlic and cook 2-3 minutes more. Add the tofu and cook, stirring frequently for 5 minutes.

Add 1 cup of the tomatoes, ¼ cup of water, and the cider vinegar. Cover and cook over low heat for 30 minutes. Add the raisins, capers, and olives and cook 15 minutes more.*

Fill the pepper halves with the tofu mixture. Pour remaining ½ cup of chopped tomatoes and ¼ cup of water into the empty sauté pan. Stir to combine and place the pepper halves into the pan. Cover loosely with foil and roast for 30 minutes (adding more water if needed) or until peppers are soft when pierced with a small knife.

*OPTION: You can serve the dish over rice after Step 3. If filling peppers, omit cooking for 15 minutes as described in Step 3 and just fill peppers to finish cooking in the oven.

ROASTED CAULIFLOWER AND POTATOES WITH TOASTED QUINOA AND AN AVOCADO/TOFU SAUCE

I'm pretty obsessed with Cauliflower. I like it raw, boiled, in rice form, and especially as the star of a roasted veggie medley. In this dish, the cauliflower shines and is accompanied with yummy roasted red potatoes, toasted quinoa underneath, and a rich and creamy avocado tofu sauce on top. The sauce can be kept in the fridge and used for other savory dishes or as a marinade for any protein you are cooking. While there are a few cooking components to making the dish, it's quite simple and you can make a double batch of the vegetables to use in salads or soups for the following few days.

Ingredients:

½ package of silken tofu
1 avocado
juice of one lime
¼ cup black beans
1 small onion
2 garlic cloves
whole cauliflower
1 cup small red potatoes
1 tbsp red wine vinegar
2 tsp plus 2 tbsp olive oil
½ cup of water
Pinch of chili powder or cayenne pepper or paprika
Salt & pepper, to taste
1 cup quinoa
Cilantro for sauce and for garnish

Method:

Veggies:

Preheat your oven to 400°F.

Rinse and core your whole cauliflower, pulling it into florets and place on a baking sheet. Add your red potatoes. Toss vegetables in 2 tsp of olive oil and salt and pepper to taste. Bake for 45 minutes

Meanwhile, cut up a clove of garlic and a small onion and sweat in a hot sauté pan with 1 tbsp of olive oil until translucent. Add salt and pepper and a pinch of chili powder

Quinoa:

While the veggies are roasting, make your quinoa according to the directions on the container. Generally, 2 cups of water is required to 1 cup of quinoa. I like to toast the quinoa first in a dry sauce pan for extra flavor. Add water and a pinch of salt. Cook for 15 minutes until water is absorbed.

Sauce:

In a blender, combine 1 avocado, the juice of one lime, ½ box of silken tofu, the red wine vinegar, water, the sautéed onions and garlic, 1 teaspoon of cilantro leaves (or parsley), chili powder, 1 tablespoon of olive oil, garlic clove, 1/3 cup black beans, salt, pepper, and blend until smooth. Add more salt if necessary.

To serve:

Place the quinoa in a shallow bowl and add the roasted vegetables on top. Pour on as much or as little sauce to accompany it and garnish with cilantro. Enjoy!

BLACK BEAN SOUP

Serves 4
Recipe by: Arlene Jacobs

Ingredients:
2 tbsp extra virgin olive oil
1 onion, diced
1 green pepper, diced
3 large garlic cloves, 2 chopped, 1 smashed
2-19 oz cans black beans with their liquid
3 sprigs thyme
1 bay leaf
1 tsp cumin
½ tsp oregano
Pinch hot pepper flakes
1 tsp red wine vinegar

Method:
In a large sauté pan over medium-high heat, sauté the onions
and peppers until beginning to soften, about three minutes. Lower
the heat and add the 2 chopped garlic cloves and cook gently for
about two minutes more.

Add the black beans and their liquid, thyme, bay leaf, cumin,
oregano, and hot pepper flakes. Add two cups water. Bring to a
boil, reduce heat to low, and continue to cook for about 20 minutes or until a full flavor develops. Add more water if necessary
and adjust seasonings.

....

6 STEPS TO FEEL BADASS IN YOUR BATHING SUIT

My *loving* response to many participants who expressed their hatred for wearing bathing suits:

Find a bathing suit that fits your unique body and style. Make sure it is comfortable and is the correct size.

Recognize and acknowledge that you feel like people may be looking at you and/or making judgements. Ask yourself, *Is this true? Or is it a story I'm making up because of how I feel about myself?*

Get in the water. We are all weightless in water and the sensory experience can help us feel embodied—one of the ways we can improve our body image.

Stand at the pool or beach for a moment in complete mindfulness and presence. Notice the thought bubbles; just notice how your body feels and where you are holding tension, ambivalence, or stress. Breathe through that and recite a positive mantra. "I am worthy as I am." "My body is meant to do amazing things." "I will not let shame or fear hold me back for what I want to do in my life." Or make up your own.

Take a minute to notice other people at the pool or beach. Notice how we are all interconnected and how we all feel the same concerns, insecurities, and self-judgements. Most people are too wrapped up in their own body concerns to be worrying or judging you. Seriously. Remember that. We all have our stories. You're allowed to let go of yours.

Take a minute to compliment at least two people. Complimenting others is a gift to them, but also to you. It doesn't have to be about that person's looks or their bathing suit. It could be about how well they are managing watching three kids at the pool or how nice their beach bag is or for their taste in music. Whatever. Give yourself a gift by making someone else's day.

....

JOURNAL QUESTIONS

When was the first time you noticed you had an opinion of your body? What was that opinion? How old were you?

_____

_____

_____

_____

_____

_____

_____

Do you remember an incident or experience where someone made a comment about your appearance that had a lasting impression on you? Write about that experience and how it shaped you.

_____

_____

_____

_____

_____

_____

_____

_____

_____

_____

What is one or more parts of your body that you love and appreciate?

_____

_____

_____

_____

_____

What is one part of your body that you dislike or are uncomfortable with?

_____

_____

_____

_____

_____

Journal about when you feel most comfortable in your skin (in certain clothing, during sex, while running, etc.).

_____

_____

_____

_____

_____

_____

_____

_____

_____

_____

Journal about when you least feel comfortable in your skin.

Write a letter to your body. What would you say to it?

_____

_____

_____

_____

_____

_____

_____

_____

_____

_____

Have your body write a letter back to you. What would its response back to you be?

_____

_____

_____

_____

_____

_____

_____

_____

_____

_____

What would it take for you to love your body unconditionally?

_____

_____

_____

_____

_____

_____

_____

_____

_____

_____

Who would you be if you didn't have to worry about your exterior appearance anymore? What would you do that you're not doing now?

_____

_____

_____

_____

_____

_____

_____

_____

_____

RESOURCES

Abby Bernstein, Figurative Photography:
www.abphotoarts.com

Jenny's Signature *Unhinge the Binge* Signature Course
jenny-eden.teachable.com/p/unhingethebinge/

Join Jenny Berk in learning some basic, yet poignant and actionable steps to slow down while eating, making more mindful choices and learning to savor your food again. This proven method to end binge, emotional and stress eating has had people focusing their energy more on living their lives versus obsessing about food and weight. Jenny will walk you through basics such as using mindfulness and planning to make food choices, how to own the decision to eat and how to savor each bite to optimize pleasure, digestion and overall well being. She will give you exercises, guided meditations, resource workbooks and homework to support you on this journey. You will also have the option to participate in live weekly online group coaching for greater support and accountability. Visit her website www.jennyedencoaching.com to learn more about her and her Beyond Weight Loss Program.

Jenny's Mindful Eating Course
jenny-eden.teachable.com/p/
my-7-day-email-course-fast-track-to-slow-eating/

Do you eat too fast? Feel like you can't figure out the difference between physical hunger and emotional hunger? Do you wonder what it would be like to know when to stop eating intuitively and trust your body? I've got solutions to all of this in my FREE 7-day email course. Learn concrete and actionable steps to be on your way to a more mindful eater and learn to have a happy and sustainable relationship with food. Includes, handouts, worksheets, checklists and more!

Body-Positive Resources:
Body Image Movement
About Face
A Beautiful Body Project
The Body Positive
Beauty Redefined
About that Curvy Life
Be Nourished
A Year Without Mirrors
Sarah Berneche

Facebook Groups:
Curvy Confidence with Natalie Baack
Taryn Brumfitt fan page
Body Love Wellness
Break the Rules: Body Positive and Anti-Diet Community with Summer Innanen

Podcasts:
The Love, Food Podcast
Food Psych Podcast
The F*ck It Diet Radio
Body Bliss
Psychology of Eating Podcast
The Everyday Woman Podcast (I'm featured on this one – episode #5)
Fearless Rebelle Radio
Let It Out with Katie Dalebout

MEDA: Multi-Service Eating Disorders Association
Boston, MA
medainc.org

NEDA: National Eating Disorders Association
nationaleatingdisorders.org

ABOUT THE AUTHOR

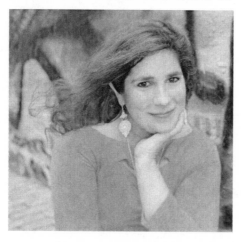

Jenny Eden Berk received her Master's Degree from the University of Pennsylvania in psychological services. She is a certified Eating Psychology Coach, mindful eating instructor, and health and wellness blogger. Jenny earned her certificate from the Institute for the Psychology of Eating in 2015 and her MB-Eat certificate in 2016. She is a regular contributor for The Huffington Post and Boston Mom's Blog. Jenny is the founder and owner of Jenny Eden Coaching—a practice devoted to help men, women, and teens create a more healthy and sustainable relationship with food and their body image.

Having struggled with food and weight for her entire life, Jenny has found deep peace with her relationship to food and her body, and is passionate about helping others achieve this as well. She considers herself a vegetarian foodie and loves to cook, bake, and entertain as well as practice hot yoga and kettlebell training.

You can reach Jenny by visiting her website: www.jennyedencoaching.com
or by joining her Wellness Warriors Facebook group.

CPSIA information can be obtained
at www.ICGtesting.com
Printed in the USA
LVOW11s1758150617

538254LV00002B/331/P